ISBN: 979-8-9926462-0-7
Cover design by Katherine Zitterbart
Interior layout by Katherine Zitterbart
For information, inquiries, or bulk orders, contact:
hello@kayteezee.com
Printed in the United States of America
Library of Congress Control Number: 2025903052
This book is intended for informational and educational purposes only. The author and publisher disclaim any liability in connection with the use of the material contained herein.

This book is intended for informational and educational purposes only. It is not a substitute for professional medical, psychological, or therapeutic advice, diagnosis, or treatment. The author and publisher make no representations or warranties regarding the accuracy, applicability, or completeness of the contents of this book.

Readers are encouraged to consult with a qualified healthcare professional before making any decisions based on the information contained herein. The author and publisher disclaim any liability for any direct, indirect, incidental, or consequential damages arising from the use or misuse of this material.

All exercises, movements, and somatic practices described in this book are to be engaged in at the reader's discretion. If you experience discomfort, pain, or distress, discontinue the activity and seek appropriate professional guidance.

By reading this book, you acknowledge and agree that the responsibility for your well-being remains solely with you.

About the Author

Katherine Zitterbart is a **Neidan practitioner, media theorist, and architect of embodied cognition.** A **fraternal twin** raised in a household of musicians and academics, she developed an early fluency in **patterns—both in sound and in thought.** She invented her own symbolic language before mastering grammar and was introduced to **Taoism at 11 and theoretical physics at 13.**

Katie's work bridges **Chinese medicine, cognitive neuroscience, and trauma-informed embodiment**, and she's been working with bodies and breath for more than 35 years.

In **2019**, she survived a **stroke that should have killed her.** In 2020, she was diagnosed with **Stage 3 Breast Cancer** and endured treatment **in total isolation at the height of the COVID-19 pandemic.** Cut off from external support, she rebuilt her nervous system **from the inside out,** developing a framework that reorients **somatics, cognition, and perception beyond supremacy-based systems.**

This is not a model of control. **It is a model of resonance.**

Her philosophy—**"Disrupt Supremacy at the Machine-Language Level"**—emerged as both a survival strategy and a structural intervention. The result is **ZitterbartEscherBach**—a system built not on hierarchy, but on **loops, tensegrity, and lived experience.**

A Note from Katie –

Please approach this as though each page is an invitation into curiosity and contemplation. There is plenty of science, methodologies, and exercises through ought. I've also included QR Codes to other media that will help you if you want to explore further. There are no paywalls. You have access because you are reading this ☺ . We are to open doors in this Work

.

My use of Large Language Models (LLMs)

I've been contemplating machine intelligence since the 1980s. It was my first major, and I was among the world's first humans to design for e-commerce at the point of exchange. I have media training by the inventor of the CD-Rom, Michael Gosney. My approach to digital is specific and rooted in Buckminster Fuller Logic.

All of which is to say, I have used LLMs in Physics, Linguistics, and TCM to ensure accuracy in my mapping and to do things like make me tables.

The framework is fully of my design. It is based on the Carl Sagan Koan: "If you want to bake an apple pie from scratch, you must first invent the universe."

Chad (my name for AI) has also assisted in typing, as I have significant impairment due to lymphedema in my dominant arm. **The mappings in my model are unique in spacetim**e. I modeled 100% of this on paper and through art before I put any of it in the machine. My approach has been ontological and rooted in my own lived experience and the decades' study and contemplation of nonduality through the lens of three.

IF YOU WANT TO BAKE AN APPLIE PIE
FROM SCRATCH, YOU MUST FIRST
INVENT THE UNIVERSE - SAGAN

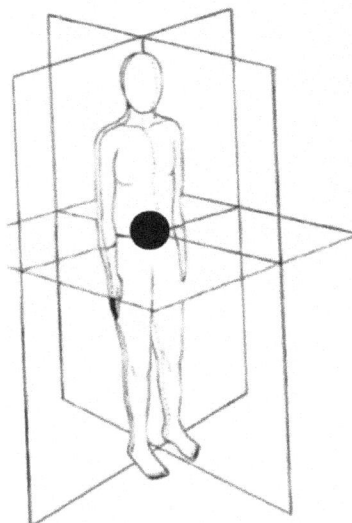

2019 STROKE
2020 BC
2023 BUILD A UNIVERSE

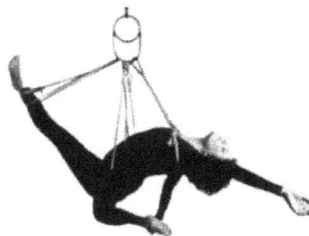

Structure / TOC

Throughout this resource are charts, tables, and QR Codes to Media.

In Service,

Katie

GOT TRAUMA?

REGULATION   RESONANCE

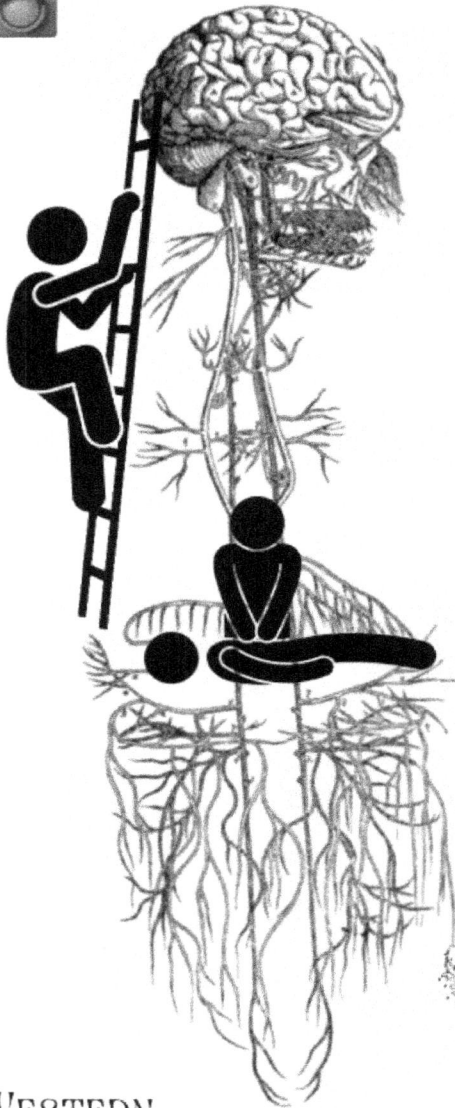

WESTERN
MEDICINE
LOGIC

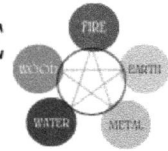

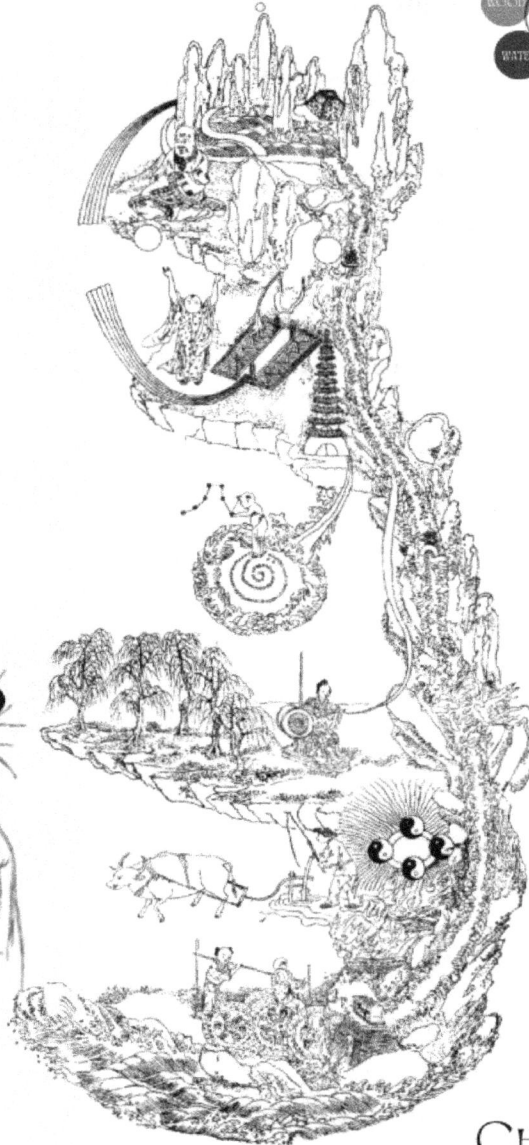

CHINESE
MEDICINE
LOGIC

The Tao That Can Be Named Is Not the Tao

This is the first lesson of Taoism and the only law. The moment we try to define something completely; we lose what it is.

"You are already inside the system."

You don't have to build it, name it, or prove it.

Your body, your breath, the weight of your awareness in space—**this is the system**. It has always been here.

This book is not an attempt to impose a new model. It is an **invitation to notice** what has already been moving beneath the surface—within you, within culture, within the living structures of the cosmos.

This is a book of **resonance, not force**. It does not ask you to change, fix, or control. It asks you to **pay attention**.

This book uses Dao and Tao interchangeably.

This Book Works Whether You Read it in Order or Not

It is impossible to out into writing what can only be experienced. Because this maps to the Brain and Body Systems, it's immediately somatic. Neuroaffective Somatics is the body aspect of a larger frame: ZitterbartEscherBach, which is based on Newtonian, Relative, and Quantum Physics.

Growth During Chaos

Rather than focusing on trauma as damage, Neuroaffective Somatics approaches it as **a process of re-patterning**—one that can be understood through the **mechanics of Chinese Medicine** (Chace 2021), aligned with **cognitive and affective neuroscience** (Panksepp and Biven 2012). Healing is not about "going back to normal"—it is about moving forward into a new configuration of self, with deeper coherence and resonance.

Taoist Inner Alchemy (Neidan) predates acupuncture by thousands of years (Pregadio 2019). In this book, we work with **the ancient maps of transformation**—not as historical artifacts, but as living frameworks for re-organizing **the nervous system, the body, and our relationship to time, lineage, and space.**

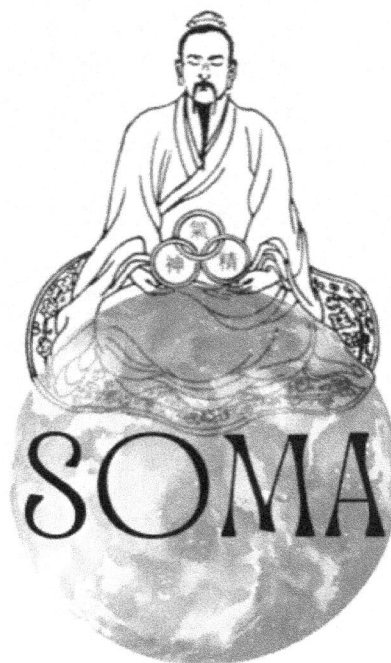

The Tai Chi (Yin-Yang) symbol at the center of the Bagua represents YOU, the practitioner.

- You are the point of balance **between inherited patterns (lineage, Jing)** and **your reach toward the cosmos (Shen, spirit).**
- You are the one **choosing how to engage with this model**—not as a passive observer but as an active participant in your own transformation.

Decoding the Symbol

The Circle around the image is called WUJI – The Great Void – so it's a bit ironic. The boundary of the symbol of yin and yang represents all that was before anything existed

The White Area is Yang
The Black area is Yin

You'll note that there is a dot of black in the white and a dot of white in the black – this is to indicate that nothing is ever completely yin or yang – there is always movement between and among them. They are related – they are not in opposition.

You might also notice that the curvature of where yin and yang come together within the symbol is reminiscent of a sine curve – a continuous wave – again showing the movement between and among yin and yang

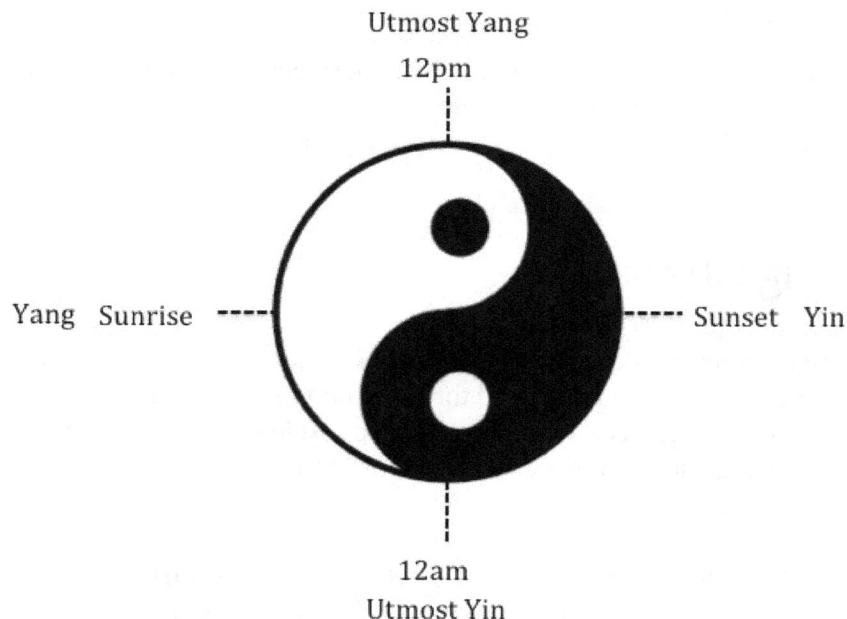

Utmost Yang

12pm

Yang Sunrise ----   ---- Sunset Yin

12am

Utmost Yin

Context is Key

A thing is Yin or Yang only within the context in which it is considered. Remember – these are qualities, not quantities. There isn't a point at which Yin becomes Yang. Can you identify the exact moment in a day when darkness becomes light? At which exact point does a leader shift from ordering to enrolling? At what temperature does it become 'cold'?

If you sit and contemplate, you'll note that all of this is relative and dependent on context.

Is 65 Degrees Yin or Yang? Well, the answer to that depends upon where and when you are:

	Yin	Yang
Temperature during Summer		
In New England	65	85
At the South Pole	-30	65

From Regulation to Resonance: Shen as the Fluid Piece

If **Yin-Yang represents polarity**, then **Shen represents coherence**—the intelligence that allows for **resonance instead of mere regulation.**

- **Regulation stops at Qi** → It focuses on managing nervous system states, controlling energy.
- **Resonance moves into Shen** → It recognizes that true regulation is not control, but alignment with the **field of relationships** that the meridians describe.

When Shen is fully expressed, **the body does not just "return to baseline"—it refines its capacity for perception, attunement, and relational depth**.

This is why **Chinese Medicine does not separate nervous system function from consciousness.** The two are one process, moving along meridian pathways, constantly shaping and reshaping experience.

In Neuroaffective Somatics: The Soma is the Portal

Neuroaffective Somatics, which is my label, is **a Soma-centered model** that integrates **neuroscience, affective science, Chinese Medicine, and somatic intelligence** to support **nervous system health, emotional resilience, and embodied awareness.**

Healing **does not happen by managing state—it happens through the Soma.**

- Through the Soma → To the Self.
- Through the Soma → To the Spirit.
- Through the Soma → To the Planet.

At its core, this framework **rejects dominance-based approaches.** Rather than trying to **regulate** the nervous system as an endpoint, it **deepens attunement to the Soma—** recognizing that all physiological states are **responses to gravitational, environmental, and social forces.**

Neuroaffective Somatics **is not a repackaging of existing somatic models.** It is a **direct response to:**

- **The limitations of Polyvagal Theory and its alignment with the DSM.**
- **Cultural appropriation in Western somatic spaces, particularly in "Skinny White Girl Yoga."**
- **The rigidity of Dialectical Behavioral Therapy (DBT), which reframes logic fallacies as cognitive distortions.**

This framework is built on decades of experience in **movement-based traditions,** including the **Krishnamacharya and Ghosh lineages of yoga,** while **fully prioritizing Traditional Chinese Medicine (TCM) and Neidan (Taoist Inner Alchemy).**

The goal is **not to impose another rigid system.** Instead, it **opens a larger field for clinicians and patients** to move beyond **binary thinking**—beyond "Am I doing it right or not?"

Neuroaffective Somatics **departs from psychiatric regulation models** that assume healing = **returning to social engagement** (Polyvagal Theory, DSM-based psychiatric frameworks). Instead, it aligns with **biological and medical models** that recognize:

- Fascia, tensegrity, and gravity as fundamental forces in human health.
- The nervous system as an orienting system rather than a regulation system.
- Somatic intelligence as a process of resonance, not control.

Aligned to Trauma-Informed Virtues & Cultural Competence

Neuroaffective Somatics is built on a foundation of lived experience. Healing is not a theoretical construct—it is shaped by **culture, history, and personal narrative**. A trauma-informed approach must recognize that **nervous system regulation cannot be separated from context**.

Trauma-informed care recognizes that healing is not just an individual journey—it is a relational, cultural, and systemic process. Each of these core virtues aligns with the **SAMHSA trauma-informed principles** while also offering a **dual perspective**:

- **Regulation Meaning** → How the virtue supports nervous system regulation, moving from defense into safety.
- **Resonance Meaning** → How the virtue extends beyond self-regulation into relational and environmental attunement, fostering deep, embodied healing. (SAMHSA, 2014)

1. Safety → The Nervous System Cannot Shift Out of Defense Mode Without It

Perspective	Meaning & Application
	The autonomic nervous system (ANS) governs survival responses. If the body perceives ongoing threat—real or perceived—it remains
Regulation Meaning	trapped in fight, flight, freeze, or fawn. Without safety, healing cannot occur.
	Safety is not just internal; it is relational. Co-regulation between self
Resonance Meaning	and environment is crucial. Humans thrive when safety is **felt, acknowledged, and mirrored** in relationships.
	Safety is not just a feeling—it is a **gravitational event**. Chronic defense states create upward tension—elevated shoulders, shallow
Neuroaffective Benefit	breath, lack of ground contact. Somatic descent (feeling weight, diaphragmatic breathing, proprioceptive awareness) restores safety.

2. Trustworthiness & Transparency → Healing Cannot Happen Through Coercion

Perspective	Meaning & Application
Regulation Meaning	The nervous system perceives **inconsistency as danger**. When messages, environments, or practitioners feel unpredictable, the body remains in hypervigilance. Transparency settles the system.
Resonance Meaning	Trust is not just personal—it is a **shared field of coherence**. A practitioner does not "heal" a client but establishes **stability and clarity**, allowing the client's nervous system to entrain into safety.
Neuroaffective Benefit	Trust is encoded through **sensorimotor rhythms**. Chronic unpredictability maintains **bracing patterns** in the fascia. Transparency in healing work allows the body to shift from **reflexive contraction to adaptability**.

3. Peer Support → Shared Experience is Medicine

Perspective	Meaning & Application
Regulation Meaning	**Isolation increases nervous system dysregulation.** The body's survival mechanisms evolved for **connection**—healing in community signals safety.
Resonance Meaning	Healing does not come from a **single truth or teacher** but through **shared stories and lived experience**. Peer support prevents hierarchy and fosters belonging.
Neuroaffective Benefit	**Shared experience organizes the body spatially.** Sensorimotor mirroring (breath, posture, micro-movements) allows the nervous system to shift state **without conscious effort**. Fascia **responds to presence**, altering tension patterns through **relational attunement**.

4. Collaboration & Mutuality → Healing Requires Shared Power

Perspective	Meaning & Application
Regulation Meaning	**Hierarchical models mirror trauma**, reinforcing powerlessness. Mutual collaboration **restores agency**, allowing healing to be participatory rather than imposed.
Resonance Meaning	**Power is not removed—it is distributed.** True transformation happens through **mutual attunement**, where both practitioner and client **co-regulate** the process.
Neuroaffective Benefit	Gravity is a **shared force**. In hierarchical structures, bodies contract or yield. In **collaborative healing**, the body reorganizes through **reciprocal movement, weight distribution, and adaptive resilience**.

5. Empowerment, Voice & Choice → The Nervous System Must Learn That It Has Agency

Perspective	Meaning & Application
Regulation Meaning	Trauma **teaches the nervous system that it is powerless.** Healing must **restore autonomy,** allowing a person to shift between **contraction and release on their own terms.**
Resonance Meaning	**Self-expression is vibrational.** When one person **finds their voice**, it shifts the energy of **relationships, communities, and cultural systems.**
Neuroaffective Benefit	**Agency is a sensorimotor function.** Fascia responds to **perceived control over movement.** Trauma restricts motion—**locked joints, shallow breath, limited spatial engagement.** Restoring **somatic adaptability** restores agency.

6. Cultural, Historical, and Gender Awareness → Trauma is Inherited, Systemic, and Relational

Perspective	Meaning & Application
Regulation Meaning	The nervous system is **shaped by lived experience and ancestral imprints.** Epigenetics shows trauma **transmits across generations,** meaning healing must include **personal, cultural, and systemic layers.**
Resonance Meaning	Healing is incomplete without **acknowledging the body's historical and cultural context.** A trauma-informed approach **does not erase differences—it acknowledges them.**
Neuroaffective Benefit	Trauma manifests **spatially—as postural rigidity, movement restriction, and gravitational compression.** Healing requires **sensorimotor recalibration— restoring full spatial range, presence, and gravitational ease.**

The Polyvagal Theory & Nervous System Regulation

I have trained extensively with Bessel vanDer Kolk, Peter Levine, and Stephen Porges, the world's leading experts on trauma. This section is based on my training with them my opinions about their work is based on lived experience.

ESSENTIAL POLYVAGAL CONCEPTS

The Polyvagal Theory is based on the idea that the vagus nerve, which is a vital part of the autonomic nervous system, has a crucial role in regulating the body's response to stress and ensuring a sense of safety. The autonomic nervous system is made up of two branches: the sympathetic nervous system and the parasympathetic nervous system. The sympathetic nervous system is responsible for the "fight or flight" response, while the parasympathetic nervous system promotes "rest and digest" functions. The vagus nerve has two branches, the ventral vagal complex and the dorsal vagal complex, which further influence the parasympathetic nervous system.

The 3 Nervous System 'States' are Hyper-Aroused (Fight/Flight), Hyper-Aroused (Freeze Fawn Appease), and Window of Tolerance - Social Engagement Network

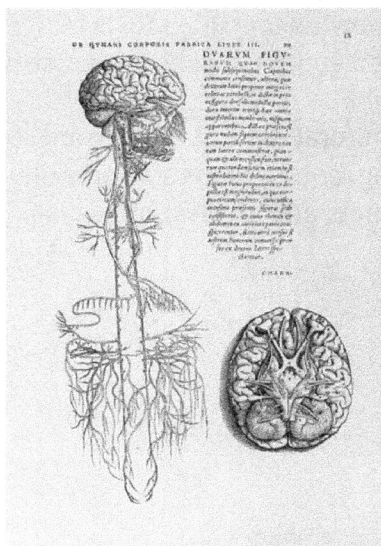

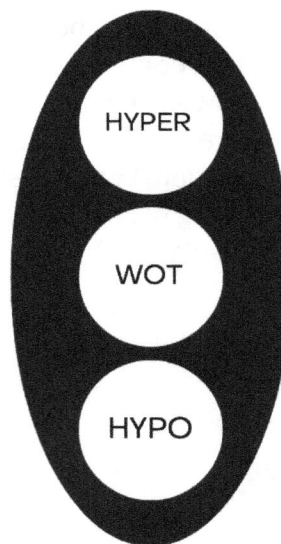

Katherine Zitterbart, MA IBOSP 617-543-9642 hello@kayteezee.com   KAYTEEZEE.COI

Polyvagal Theory (PVT) is one of the most widely used frameworks for understanding the nervous system in trauma work. Developed by Dr. Stephen Porges, it explains how our autonomic nervous system shifts between states of **safety, danger, and shutdown**—and how these shifts influence our ability to connect, respond, and recover from stress (Porges, 2011).

The core of PVT is the **Vagus nerve** which regulates heart rate, digestion, and social engagement. Unlike earlier models, which divided the nervous system into simple "fight-or-flight" (sympathetic) and "rest-and-digest" (parasympathetic) responses, PVT proposes a **three-tiered hierarchy of states**:

The Three States of the Autonomic Nervous System

- **Ventral Vagal (Social Engagement) → Regulation & Connection**
  - The body feels **safe, calm, and open** to social interaction.
  - Breath is steady, heart rate is balanced, and the nervous system is flexible.
  - This state is often seen as the "goal" of nervous system health.
- **Sympathetic (Mobilization) → Fight or Flight**
  - The body is **activated**, primed for action, movement, or defense.
  - Heart rate speeds up, muscles tense, focus narrows.
  - This is often labeled as "stress" or "anxiety," but it is also **the energy that drives momentum and motivation**.
- **Dorsal Vagal (Immobilization) → Shutdown & Collapse**
  - The body **withdraws, slows down, and disconnects**.
  - This can look like **dissociation, fatigue, numbness, or a freeze response**.
  - In extreme cases, it leads to **shutdown, hypoarousal, or dissociative states**.

PVT presents these three states as a **ladder**:

- At the top, **ventral vagal safety** allows for social engagement and regulation.
- In the middle, **sympathetic activation** mobilizes the body for fight or flight.
- At the bottom, **dorsal vagal shutdown** pulls the system into conservation and collapse (Porges, 2011)

State	Nervous System Function	Somatic & Emotional Experience
Ventral Vagal (Safety & Social Engagement)	Co-regulation, relational openness	Calm, connected, expressive, adaptable
Sympathetic (Mobilization: Fight-or-Flight)	Activation, defense, movement	Alert, anxious, reactive, mobilized
Dorsal Vagal (Immobilization: Freeze & Shutdown)	Withdrawal, conservation	Numb, disconnected, fatigued, collapsed

According to this model, **regulation** means moving up the ladder—away from collapse, through activation, and into connection.

The Window of Tolerance

Polyvagal-based therapies often use the **Window of Tolerance**, a model introduced by Dr. Dan Siegel, to describe the range in which the nervous system can function without becoming overwhelmed.

- Inside the window, the nervous system is **regulated**. Stress is manageable, emotions are fluid, and thinking is clear.
- Outside the window, the nervous system becomes **dysregulated**.
  - **Hyperarousal (fight/flight):** Overwhelm, panic, anxiety, anger.
  - **Hypoarousal (freeze/shutdown):** Numbness, dissociation, exhaustion.
- The goal of regulation is to **bring the system back inside the window** so it can function optimally.

This model has shaped an entire generation of nervous system work. It's a powerful tool, but it is incomplete.

In the **Polyvagal framework, dysregulation** is seen as an autonomic failure—a sign that the body has not learned how to **self-soothe and return to safety.**

Cultural Gaps in Polyvagal Theory

Polyvagal Theory presents itself as a universal model of the nervous system, but **whose nervous system does it describe?** The idea of **regulation** is built on assumptions about **what a regulated body looks like**, and those assumptions are not neutral.

The **dominant lens in psychiatric and nervous system research is white, male, Western, neurotypical, and able-bodied.** The **behaviors that are pathologized**—or labeled as "dysregulated"—are often those that fall outside of this narrow window (Washington, 2006).

Regulation as a Culturally Conditioned Standard

In Polyvagal Theory, a **regulated nervous system** is typically described as:

- **Calm, pleasant facial expression**
- **Even, measured tone of voice**
- **Steady breath and heart rate**
- **Comfort with direct eye contact**
- **A balance of assertiveness and receptivity**

But these **markers of regulation are not universal**—they are conditioned by **race, gender, neurodivergence, and cultural norms.**

- **Black individuals** are more likely to be labeled **schizophrenic** when exhibiting sensory overwhelm, dissociation, or emotional intensity that would be recognized as **autism or PTSD** in a white body.
- **Women** expressing mood shifts, dissociation, or emotional shutdown are more likely to be diagnosed with **bipolar disorder** than **C-PTSD**—despite trauma often being the underlying factor.
- **Indigenous, Black, and Latinx children** are disproportionately diagnosed with **behavioral disorders** rather than being recognized as experiencing **trauma or neurodivergence.**
- **Neurodivergent individuals** (especially autistic people) may not show "social engagement" in a way that aligns with **Polyvagal Theory's ventral vagal standard**, leading to misinterpretations of their **nervous system state**.

]

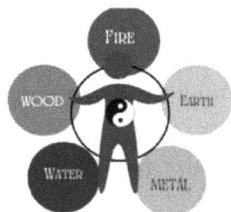

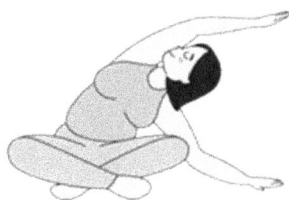

DON'T REGULATE - RESONATE!

EXTRAORDINARY YIN

NERVOUS SYSTEM RESONANCE
AND FASCIA FORMATIONS

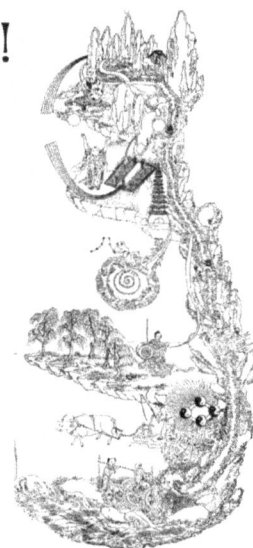

The Medical Model is Fixated on Control

Western trauma frameworks—including Polyvagal Theory—often operate within a dominance-based model, assuming that a nervous system in control is a healthy nervous system. This approach medicalizes the natural responses of marginalized bodies while failing to account for the environmental and systemic factors shaping those responses (Washington 2006; Kendi 2016; Manne 2020; Menakem 2021).

For example:

- The history of medicine is steeped in systemic biases that disproportionately pathologize Black bodies (Washington 2006). "Cultural narratives about trauma and dysregulation are shaped by structures of power, not just by physiology (Kendi 2016; Manne 2020).
- A **queer or gender-nonconforming person** who learns to mask their identity in certain spaces might experience **somatic tension, digestive issues, and dissociation**—but their nervous system adaptations are rarely understood through a trauma-aware, body-centered lens.

If **regulation** is defined only by **Western, white, neurotypical standards of social engagement**, it will fail to recognize the **lived experience of anyone outside that framework.**

This is why **resonance matters more than regulation.**

Resonance in the Neuroaffective Model

Neuroaffective Somatics is based on fully non-invasive Chinese Medicine through the Inner Alchemy that informs it. I've used my extensive background in ontology, software design, and media theory to accurately map concepts across disciplines.

Acupuncture's origins are deeply tied to the philosophy of Huang Di. The story goes that Huang Di, as a wise ruler, sought to understand the mysteries of life, health, and disease. Observing the natural world and humanity's interaction with it, he discovered that certain patterns in nature mirrored the human body's processes. He believed that the body's energy system (qi) could be influenced through specific points to restore balance and health. His insights, likely drawn from early observations of injury, touch, and pressure, were refined into acupuncture techniques.

"When we talk about the five elements, we are discussing the dynamics of the creative and control cycles, the changes of excess and deficiency, and so forth. By understanding the principles underlying these changes, we can apply them to disease progression." – (Unschuld, 2011 p 25)

Huang Di (The Yellow Emperor) and Acupuncture

One of Huang Di's most significant contributions is his association with traditional Chinese medicine (TCM), especially acupuncture and moxibustion. While it is unlikely that Huang Di personally "created" acupuncture, he is symbolically connected to its origins because of his association with the foundational text of Chinese medicine, the **Huangdi Neijing**, or "The Yellow Emperor's Inner Canon" (Unschuldm 2011).s

This text, written between 2,000 and 2,500 years ago, is attributed to conversations between Huang Di and his ministers, particularly his chief physician, Qi Bo. In these dialogues, they discuss the theories of health, illness, and the human body in relation to natural forces like yin and yang, the Five Elements (Wood, Fire, Earth, Metal, Water), and qi (vital energy). Acupuncture is presented in this text as a therapeutic technique to balance qi flow through the body's meridians (energy pathways) by stimulating specific points on the skin with needles.

In the **Huangdi Neijing (Yellow Emperor's Inner Canon)** and the **Dao De Jing**, leadership is not about dominance—it is about **attunement**. The text does not present the emperor as one who controls, but as one who listens, perceives, and **teaches through presence rather than force.**

This understanding marks the **transition from regulation to resonance.**

Regulation seeks to establish order—to manage energy, to balance excess and deficiency, to maintain harmony through cycles of restriction and generation. But **resonance** asks something deeper:

- **How does one align with the Dao rather than impose upon it?**
- **How do we not just self-regulate, but enter into coherence with the living world?**
- **How do we embody transformation rather than merely attempt to direct it?**

The **generation and restriction cycles** of the **Five Elements** are not just models of balance; they are **archetypes of leadership.** They demonstrate that true guidance is not about **controlling outcomes** but about **understanding natural relationships** (Unschuld, 2011).

Neuroaffective Somatics is Rooted In Neidan: Taoist Inner Alchemy

As Yoga, Neuroaffective Somatics is based on my experience with **Neidan (內丹)**, or **Internal Alchemy**. Neidan is among the most esoteric of practices and is the alchemy that TCM is based on. Almost all of my exposure in Neidan originated with a living human. My mother introduced me to the Tao te Ching at 11, and when I learned about Memetics from the philosopher/physicist Douglas Hofstadter, my unrecognized autistic brain found a meta-system. **Shen** is the word TCM uses for 'spirit' of the law. I've historically referred to it as 'the third factor'. What I'm doing here is creating transparency for you. We are to guide in this system – not create barriers.

The Three Virtues: Compassion, Moderation, Humility

Taoism centers 3 Virtues, which create the ethical foundation for both Huangdi **Neijing** (Acupuncture) and the **Dao De Jing (Philosophy):**

1. **Compassion (Ci, 慈)** – The desire for less suffering.
2. **Moderation (Jian, 儉)** – Restraint to avoid extremes, knowing that excess and deficiency are both disturbances in flow.
3. **Humility (Bu Gan Wei Tian Xia Xian, 不敢为天下先)** – One does not and cannot perceive all things.

This last point is crucial. The **Yellow Emperor's Inner Canon is explicit:** perception is always **partial**—we are not separate from the Dao, so we cannot command it. We are encouraged towards Natural Law, rather than Man-Made Law. This balances the rigidity of the Medical Model.

Neidan teaches that the body itself **is the landscape through which we learn to attune to the greater field.** By contemplating **Soma as Species** rather than as an isolated person, **we shift from individual survival to collective resonance.** (Pregadio, 2019)

- Instead of seeking control, we cultivate coherence.
- Instead of imposing will, we refine perception.
- Instead of assuming authority, we allow the natural intelligence of life to reveal itself.

This is not an abstraction—**it is a lived practice.** From the microcosm of the breath to the macrocosm of celestial movement, **Neidan does not ask us to "fix" anything—it asks us to perceive more deeply, to participate more fully, to refine more skillfully.**

Another Way of Knowing

Neuroaffective Somatics is **the result of a lifetime of applying the principles of Neidan** to the lived experience of human perception, trauma, and transformation. I've approached this design as though I was creating a garden of knowing, and how would I plant the initial seeds, such that the favor was always to Life…. The result is a mapping of this highly esoteric system to the human body. A whole new way to contemplate soma.

These tools are inherently neutral; as such, you can apply them within any framework. Use what works – keep the rest on the shelf.

The Bagua as a Map: A Traditional and Embodied Framework

The **Bagua (八卦)** is one of the most fundamental maps of **Daoist cosmology, natural law, and human experience**. Traditionally, it is used to:

1. **Describe the fundamental forces of nature**—each trigram represents a core **pattern of movement and transformation** (e.g., Heaven, Earth, Wind, Fire).
2. **Structure family dynamics**—the trigrams correspond to family roles (e.g., Qian ☰ as the father, Kun ☷ as the mother, Zhen ☳ as the eldest son).
3. **Illuminate the cycles of life**—the trigrams describe **human processes, emotional states, and developmental patterns**.

Trigram	Element	Direction	Family Role	Natural Image	Key Attributes
Qiān ☰	Heaven	Northwest	Father	Sky	Strength, initiative, leadership, clarity, endurance
Kun ☷	Earth	Southwest	Mother	Fertile soil	Receptivity, nourishment, patience, deep support, embodiment
Zhen ☳	Thunder	East	Eldest Son	Storm, shaking force	Activation, initiation, movement, boldness, resilience
Xùn ☴	Wind/Wood	Southeast	Eldest Daughter	Wind, gentle penetration	Flexibility, expansion, wisdom, structural balance, inheritance
Lí ☲	Fire	South	Middle Daughter	Sun, radiant energy	Illumination, transformation, wisdom, passion, ancestral memory
Kǎn ☵	Water	North	Middle Son	Deep water, abyss	Depth, emotion, reflection, adaptability, surrender
Duì ☱	Lake/Metal	West	Youngest Daughter	Open water, joy	Expression, refinement, harmony, spontaneity, communication
Gèn ☶	Mountain/Earth	Northeast	Youngest Son	Still mountain, stability	Stillness, vision, restoration, endurance, dept

Mapping the Body Systems through the Bagua

Traditional TCM attributes **Shen (spirit/consciousness)** to the **organs**, allowing us to understand **body-mind connections** not as **mechanical functions**, but as **living, relational systems** (Rossi, 2007). In this model, I've **expanded that concept beyond individual organs**. Instead, I've mapped the **Eight Extraordinary Vessels—the body's deepest currents of life energy—to the Bagua.** This aligns:

- **The body systems** with **energetic structures** rather than isolated functions.
- **The movement of Qi** with **the dynamic interactions of natural forces.**
- **The Taoist Immortals** with **the Extraordinary Vessels**, offering an **archetypal framework for transformation and embodiment.**

This approach creates a system that is:

- **Practical**—rooted in **lived experience and spatial awareness**, rather than abstraction.
- **Dynamic**—a system of **movement, transformation, and relationship**, rather than static categories.
- **Holistic**—bridging **biology, lineage, and environment** into a **single field of contemplation**.

By doing this, we mimic the way **TCM attributes Shen to the organs**, but in a **three-dimensional, embodied way**—one that acknowledges:

- **Epigenetic inheritance** (how we carry ancestral patterns).
- **Environmental influence** (how our surroundings shape our body-mind).
- **Personal cultivation** (how we refine and transform our lived experience).

Neidan (內丹) –Daoist Internal Alchemy

Neidan, or Internal Alchemy, is one of the most esoteric and profound practices within Daoist tradition. Unlike external alchemy (**Waidan**), which sought physical immortality through herbal and mineral compounds, **Neidan is an internal process of refinement**—transforming **Jing (Essence), Qi (Vital Energy), and Shen (Spirit)** into a state of harmony and deep attunement.

Within the Neuroaffective framework, Neidan provides context for Afferent/Efferent as deeply personal and specific. This practice is both **deeply personal and entirely impersonal**:

- It does not frame the **human** as an isolated entity but rather as **a species, a pattern, an unfolding expression of nature itself.**
- It is not about **strengthening the self**, but about **aligning with the natural rhythms of the universe**.
- It does not seek **control**, but rather **resonance**—learning to move with, rather than against, the fundamental forces of life.

Afferent/Efferent in the Context of Neuroaffective Somatics

Neuroaffective Somatics offers a **new way to contemplate the Eight Extraordinary Vessels and the Eight Immortals** within the **Neuroaffective Somatics framework.**

In both **neurophysiology and somatic experience**, the distinction between **afferent and efferent pathways** mirrors the relationship between **perception and action, awareness and embodiment, Shen and Jing**.

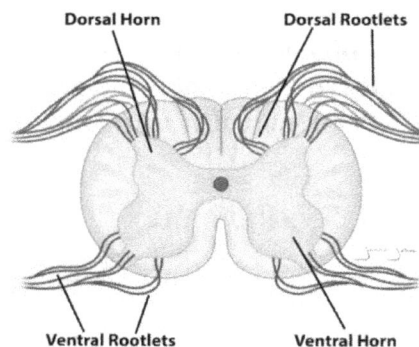

This aligns directly with **the Eight Immortals (Afferent, Shen, Dorsal)** and **the Eight Extraordinary Vessels (Efferent, Jing, Ventral)**. The afferent nervous system carries sensory input to the brain via dorsal pathways, allowing for perception and interpretation (Netter 2018).

Afferent (Dorsal, Incoming, Sensory)

- **Dorsal pathways** bring **information into the system**—they receive and interpret external and internal stimuli.
- **This is how we make meaning of experience—how we develop perception, narrative, and embodied awareness.**
- **Each Immortal represents a specific mode of perception—a unique "meme" that shapes how we interpret our world. You'll meet them later.**

Efferent (Ventral, Outgoing, Motor)

- **Ventral pathways** control **motor output, embodiment, and action**—they determine how perception translates into movement and response.
- **The Eight Extraordinary Vessels function as the structural and energetic pathways that enact what is received from the afferent perception.**
- **Each Vessel represents a specific developmental process—an embodied action that completes the loop between sensing and doing.** The Magical/Mystical: Favoring the Living Tissues

Traditional Chinese Medicine (TCM) has always been **deeply mystical**—not because it is vague, but because it recognizes the **unseen intelligence of the body**. Shen is the field through which this intelligence moves.

Contemplating Shen as Afferent: Perception, Presence, and the Living Body

From a **Neuroaffective Somatics perspective**, we contemplate **Shen as Afferent**—the way we **perceive, receive, and attune to experience.** Rather than something distant or transcendent, **Shen is what orients us toward the present moment.**

In contemplating **Shen as Afferent,** we trust that:

- **Perception itself is medicine.** To become aware of something **is already to shift it.**
- **The body organizes itself when given the right conditions.** We don't have to "force" healing—our tissues respond to **movement, breath, and presence.**
- **The Eight Extraordinary Vessels shape reality at a level beyond linear understanding.** Their effects do not have to be "proven" to be **deeply felt.**

Just as **acupuncture, Qigong, and Daoist practices trust in the body's innate capacity to heal,** so too does **Neuroaffective Somatics trust in the afferent nature of Shen—** that **awareness itself is a pathway to transformation.**

The complexity of the Neuroaffective Lens:

1. **Bridges Myth and Biology** → The Immortals and the Extraordinary Vessels are no longer separate; they are part of a **unified developmental cycle**.
2. **Aligns with Trauma Healing** → Healing is not about "fixing" the nervous system; it is about **re-experiencing developmental stages with new agency**. The Vessels provide **somatic structure**, while the Immortals provide **narrative intelligence**.
3. **Creates a Practical Contemplation Tool** → Instead of asking, "What's wrong with my Vessel?" we ask, **"How is this Immortal/Vessel pairing playing out in my life? "**

Feng Shui: Aligning the Inner & Outer Worlds

Feng Shui (风水, "Wind and Water") is the Daoist practice of **harmonizing spaces** to reflect the natural flow of Qi (vital energy). It teaches that **the environment shapes consciousness**, just as the body's energetic currents shape health (Predagio, 2016). It uses the Bagua as a way to map physical space, and it operates as the Extraordinary Map in this system.

By integrating Feng Shui principles into the somatic model, we recognize that **healing is not just internal**—it is about the relationship between:

- **Body Systems** (physiological & energetic structures).
- **The Bagua** (cosmic archetypes and environmental relationships).
- **The Practitioner** (the conscious, aware presence at the center of the system).

Tensegrity: Structure and Practice

Polyvagal Theory explains how the nervous system shifts between states, but these states do not exist in isolation—they are embedded within the body's structural and energetic framework. Stability is not just about nervous system regulation; it is about how the entire body distributes tension; processes force and maintains integrity under changing conditions. This is where tensegrity becomes essential.

Rather than a top-down system of control, the body functions as a dynamic, responsive web—where every shift in state is reflected through movement, fascia, and gravitational alignment.

Tensegrity (tensional integrity) is the fundamental **principle that allows the body to be both stable and dynamic**—not through rigidity, but through the continuous **balance of tension and compression**. **Tensegrity relies on Gravity** (Tufte 1983).

In **biotensegrity**, the body is not a structure of stacked bones and isolated muscles. Instead, it is a **web-like system where every part is interconnected**—like a suspension bridge or a geodesic dome. The **fascia**, the connective tissue that weaves through every muscle, organ, and bone, is what enables this **dynamic equilibrium**.

Why is Tensegrity Important?

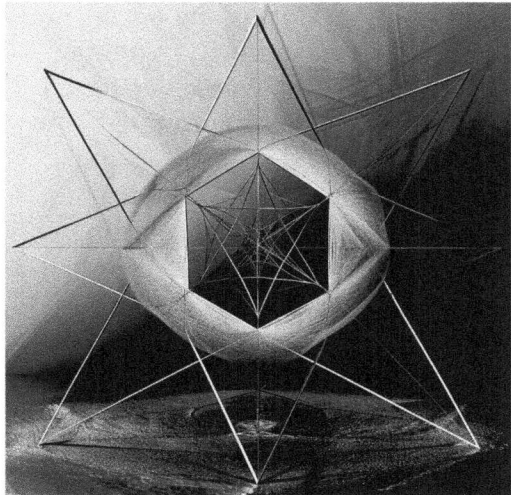

- **Elastic Strength:** Instead of resisting force, the body distributes tension **across the whole system**, allowing for effortless movement.
- **Whole-Body Coordination:** Movement isn't just about muscles—it is about how the **entire structure adjusts and adapts** in real time.
- **Resonance, Not Rigidity:** Like a well-tuned instrument, the body doesn't just "hold" a position—it **responds and flows** with pressure, weight, and environment.

Embodied Experience: Feeling Tensegrity in Action
Try this: Instead of standing "rigidly upright," imagine yourself as a **web of elastic threads**. Shift slightly. Feel how the whole system **adjusts, balances, and absorbs movement**. This is tensegrity in action.

Tensegrity = Wu-Wei = Resonance
Tensegrity is **not about control—it is about relationship**. When we move **with** the body's natural structure instead of against it, we experience **Wu-Wei—effortless action. Tensegrity is not just a mechanical principle—it is the structural embodiment of Wu-Wei.** Instead of forcing alignment, the body organizes itself **through relationship, not control.**

Just as a geodesic dome remains stable through **distributed tension**, the human body moves **most efficiently when it follows its own intrinsic patterns.** Instead of fixing posture or "holding" a state, **we follow the natural currents of flow.**

Traditional Chinese Medicine is a Tensegrity Model

Polyvagal Theory describes the **nervous system as a hierarchy of states**, moving between **social engagement, mobilization, and shutdown.** But **healing and embodied intelligence do not emerge from control—they emerge from resonance.** This is where **Traditional Chinese Medicine (TCM) provides a more dynamic, relational model—** one that moves beyond linear regulation into a **tensegrity-based understanding of the body as a fluid, adaptive system.**

TCM does not treat the nervous system as an isolated regulator. Instead, it understands **health as an ongoing negotiation between Yin and Yang, stability and movement, structure and flow.** This is the very definition of **tensegrity**—where balance is not achieved through rigidity, but through **dynamic tension and distributed forces.**

- **The Fascia as the Meridian System** → Fascia functions as **the body's primary tensegrity network**, distributing force, tension, and sensory input across the whole system. TCM's **Meridian System operates similarly**, guiding **Qi (energy) through interwoven channels** rather than through isolated pathways.
- **The Organs as Resonant Fields** → Rather than discrete biological units, the organs in TCM are understood **in relationship**—as functional networks that **support, regulate, and restrain one another in cycles of adaptation.** This mirrors how **tensegrity-based structures distribute stress across a system rather than collapsing into isolated points of failure.**
- **Jing, Chi, and Shen as Multi-Scale Adaptation** → Jing (essence) is the foundation, the **stored mass** in the tensegrity system. **Chi (energy) is the flow**, the force that allows movement and adaptation. **Shen (awareness) is the emergent pattern**, the resonance that organizes the system.

Western anatomy and trauma models often emphasize **stability through external correction—** but in **TCM and tensegrity, stability arises from intrinsic adaptability.**

- **Health is not a return to baseline—it is the ability to shift, adjust, and move fluidly between states.**
- **The body does not need to be "regulated" into stillness—it needs to be supported in its natural rhythms of expansion and contraction.**
- **Rather than "fixing" posture or movement, tensegrity-based systems allow for continuous reorganization in response to gravity, emotion, and experience.**

By shifting from **hierarchical control to relational attunement**, tensegrity and TCM provide a **functional model for embodied healing**—one that integrates **the nervous system, the fascial system, and the field of consciousness itself.**

Tensegrity of Yin and Yang : "Fixed"

At its core, **Yin and Yang are not things but processes**—interwoven movements of reality that arise from and return to the **Tao**, the undivided whole. The **Taoist worldview does not see duality as opposition, but as interplay**, where each force shapes and defines the other in a continuous dance of transformation.

This is not a static balance but a **living, breathing dynamic**—a constant unfolding where Yin contains the seed of Yang, and Yang carries the potential of Yin. To contemplate Yin and Yang in the Taoist sense is to shift away from rigid categorization and toward **an experiential understanding of how all things flow between phases of contraction and expansion, rest and motion, darkness and light.**

Wu-Wei: Power With (Shentegrity) – Fluid (Shen)

The difference between **regulation and resonance** is the difference between **control and relationship.** It is also the difference between **forcing movement** and **moving with the flow of life.**

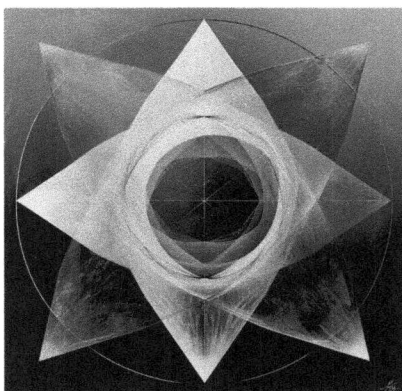

Western trauma models, including **Polyvagal Theory**, often frame **regulation** as the process of **managing the nervous system, climbing back to safety, and restoring control.** Regulation assumes the body must be **corrected**—that stability is something we must regain through effort.

In **Chinese Medicine and Daoist philosophy**, movement is **not forced—it is followed.** The nervous system is not a system of **control** but of **relationship**—it flows, adapts, cycles, and resonates. This is the heart of **Wu-Wei (無為)**—**"non-doing," or effortless action.**

To practice **Wu-Wei** is not to be passive, but to **align with the forces already moving.** Instead of trying to **dominate the nervous system into a regulated state**, we attune to **its rhythms, its tides, its natural responsiveness.**

This is **Power With**, rather than **Power Over.**

- **Regulation seeks to fix the body. Wu-Wei allows the body to self-organize.**
- **Regulation forces stability. Resonance finds harmony within change.**
- **Regulation tries to control movement. Wu-Wei moves with movement itself.**

Contemplation Suggestion: Feeling Tensegrity in Stillness

Recalling the Feeling of Buoyancy in the Womb – ZitterbartEscherBach – 2023

Take a moment to **sit or stand without forcing posture**. Instead of "holding yourself up," imagine your body as **a floating structure of elastic threads**—a web of **tension and compression, continuously adjusting to gravity.**

- Can you feel **subtle shifts in weight and balance** as you breathe?
- Notice how **stability doesn't come from rigidity, but from responsiveness**.
- Where do you sense **effort**? Where do you sense **ease**?

Now, apply **Wu-Wei**—don't try to correct anything. Simply **observe how your body self-organizes** when you stop micromanaging it.

What happens when you allow movement to arise naturally, rather than controlling it?

Biotensegrity: Fascia

Biotensegrity is the principle that **stability is not about fixed points but about dynamic tension across a whole system**. Fascia, the continuous web of connective tissue in the body, is what allows for **this adaptability, responsiveness, and integrity of movement** (Lesondak, 2017)

Where traditional models treat the body as a stack of mechanical parts, **biotensegrity reveals the body as a living, responsive structure—where every point is in relationship with every other.**

In Chinese Medicine, this principle is embedded in **Qi, the Five Elements, and the continuous interplay of expansion and contraction, rest motion, darkness and light.**

and

Tension is not rigidity. Compression is not collapse. They exist together, creating movement, responsiveness, and flow.

This is the shift from seeing the body as **fixed levers and pulleys** to understanding it as an **interwoven matrix of continuous communication.**

Before we talk about **fascia and movement,** we must first recognize **biotensegrity as the underlying field from which all movement emerges.**

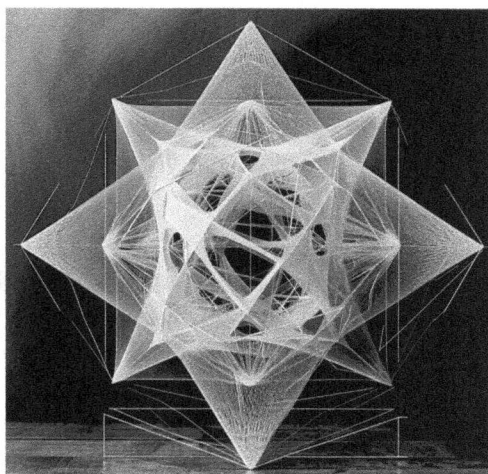

Fascia Fix: 2 Hour Masterclass and Slides

FASCIA FIX: 2 HOUR
MASTERCLASS WITH SLIDES

Living Tissue as the Unifying Medium

Traditional Chinese Medicine (TCM) does not separate **structure from function, nor perception from form**—it centers **tactility and living tissue** as the primary way to understand the body. Unlike Western anatomy, which often relies on **dissection and isolated systems**, TCM is rooted in **palpation, sensation, and the movement of Qi through a continuous, dynamic network**.

Because TCM works with **what is alive, what can be felt, and what responds to touch**, it **naturally aligns with fascia—the continuous web of connective tissue that integrates every part of the body into a single system**.

- **The meridians are not imaginary lines—they are fascial pathways.** When a practitioner works with acupuncture or bodywork, they are **not manipulating isolated nerves or muscles** but rather **influencing the entire biotensegral network through fascia.**
- **Qi itself can be understood through fascial conduction.** Fascia is both **structural and sensory**, capable of transmitting force, tension, and bioelectric signals. This explains why acupuncture points **correlate with fascial intersections**—these are places where **tensional forces converge and reorganize.**
- **Health is about dynamic adaptability, not isolated correction.** Western medicine often treats dysfunction as **a local problem**, whereas TCM sees **tissue, energy, and function as interwoven**, always responding to **gravity, movement, and environmental input.**

Biotensegrity provides the structural model that explains why TCM works. Fascia, rather than the nervous system alone, serves as the **medium of adaptation, responsiveness, and whole-body communication**. This means that every intervention in TCM—whether acupuncture, bodywork, or breathwork—is ultimately **a form of biotensegral tuning, helping the system redistribute force and restore resonance.**

Based on Gravity & Elements

While it is not groundbreaking to contemplate a human as alive, to my awareness mapping TCM onto the three Axis has not been done before. I designed this as a triple-triaxial deep neural network, with the origin at the nexus of human – the Navel. The full structure is a 9x9x9 cubist algorithm.

The Body's Three Planes: Sagittal, Coronal, Transverse

The human body moves in **three primary planes**, which reflect **different dimensions of experience and integration. Neuroaffective Somatics** aligns these planes with **embodied perception**, positioning the body in **a way that mirrors the brain—not as something to be cut into parts, but as a unified system of movement and awareness.**

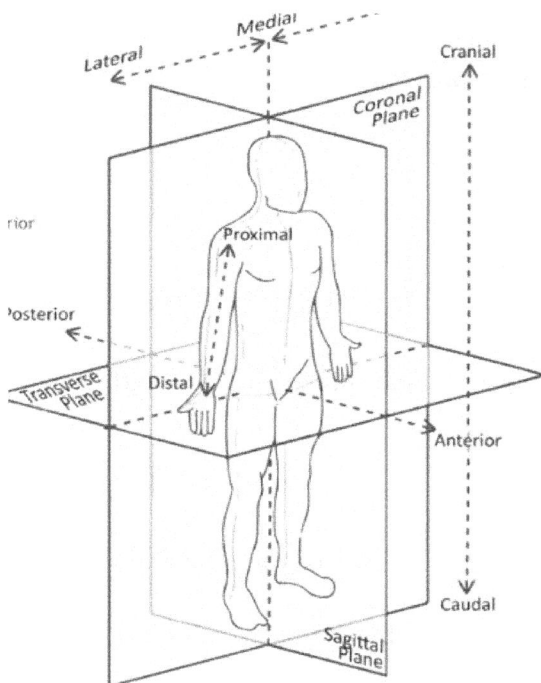

1. Sagittal Plane (Yin/Yang of Forward & Backward Movement)

- Governs **flexion and extension** (action vs. rest, fight vs. freeze).
- Most trauma models **overemphasize** this plane—focusing on **how we move toward or away from safety** but ignoring lateral and rotational dimensions.

2. Coronal Plane (Yin/Yang of Internal & Side-to-Side Movement)

- Governs **balance, relational orientation, and stability**.
- Determines **how the nervous system orients in space**, regulating **postural integrity and equilibrium**.

3. Transverse Plane (The Missing Dimension—Rotation, Integration, and Shen)

- Governs **spiral movement, depth perception, and attunement**.
- This is where **Shen enters**—allowing **integration rather than just reaction**.
- Often overlooked in traditional trauma frameworks, but **essential for true embodiment and transformation**.

These three planes **map directly to the body's sensory-motor experience** and are **deeply interwoven with the movement of Qi, the fascia system, and the Extraordinary Vessels.**

Water – The Sagittal Plane: Forward & Backward

Water is Shen—the force of perception, surrender, and deep intelligence. It governs how we **receive and process the world through movement, breath, and experience.**

Key Functions of Water (Shen in the Body)

- **Governs the nervous system and breath** – The body's ability to respond, adapt, and integrate sensory input.
- **Shapes forward and backward movement** – Moving toward experience (engagement) or pulling back (retreat).
- **Regulates perception and flow** – How we **experience time, fear, and momentum.**

Embodied Water Contemplation (Shen in Motion)

- How do you **move toward or away from experience?**
- Can you sense the **relationship between breath and movement?**
- Does your body feel **rushed, hesitant, or fluid?**

Earth – The Transverse Plane: Rotation & Integration

Earth is Jing—the foundation, the deep structure of form. It determines how we **hold, release, and integrate** movement and experience.

Key Functions of Earth (Jing in the Body)

- **Governs deep physical stability** – The core architecture of the body and its ability to hold form.
- **Shapes rotation and twisting movements** – The body's ability to weave and integrate experience.
- **Regulates embodied memory** – How we **store, process, and release tension and inherited patterns.**

Embodied Earth Contemplation (Jing in Motion)

- Can you feel how your body **twists and spirals naturally?**
- Where do you experience **fluidity vs. restriction in rotation?**
- Do you feel **centered in movement, or easily thrown off balance?**

Fire – The Coronal Plane: Side-to-Side Movement

Fire is Qi—the movement of life force through relationship, rhythm, and balance. It determines how we **interact with space, others, and self-expression.**

Key Functions of Fire (Qi in the Body)

- **Governs relational energy** – How we hold boundaries, expand, and contract in interaction.
- **Shapes side-to-side motion and weight distribution** – Balance between **internal and external forces.**
- **Regulates the body's energetic projection** – How we **express ourselves through movement and posture.**

Embodied Fire Contemplation (Qi in Motion)

- How do you experience **balance between self and world?**
- Do you feel **collapsed inward or overly expanded outward?**
- Can you sense where you **hold tension in your lateral movement?**

These axis are inherent to the TCM, and are accessed via Meridians.

Lecture and Slides introducing the Emotional Alchemy of this System

Body Wisdom: Meridians

ANTERIOR VIEW
LEFT - YIN SUPERFICIAL MERIDIANS
RIGHT - SUPERFICIAL MUSCULATURE

ARM YIN MERIDIANS & SHICHEN
LU - LUNG MERIDIAN 3 -5 AM
HT - HEART MERIDIAN 11 AM - 1 PM
LV - LIVER MERIDIAN 1 - 3 AM

LEG YIN MERIDIANS & SHICHEN
SP - SPLEEN MERIDIAN 9 - 11 AM
KD - KIDNEY MERIDIAN 5 -7 PM
PE - PERICARDIUM MERIDIAN 7 - 9 PM
CV - CONCEPTION VESSEL (CENTERLINE)

POSTERIOR VIEW
LEFT - SUPERFICIAL MUSCULATURE
RIGHT - YANG SUPERFICIAL MERIDIANS

ARM YANG MERIDIANS & SHICHEN
LI - LARGE INTESTINE MERIDIAN 5 - 7 AM
SI - SMALL INTESTINE 1 - 3 PM
TW - TRIPLE WARMER 9 - 11 PM

LEG YANG MERIDIANS & SHICHEN
ST - STOMACH MERIDIAN 7 - 9 AM
BL - BLADDER MERIDIAN 3 - 5 PM
GB - GALL BLADDER MERIDIAN 11 PM - 1 AM
GV - GOVERNING VESSEL (CENTERLINE)

LEGEND

WOOD PHASE MERIDIAN
1ST FIRE PHASE MERIDIAN
2ND FIRE PHASE MERIDIAN
EARTH PHASE MERIDIAN
METAL PHASE MERIDIAN
WATER PHASE MERIDIAN
PRIME VESSEL

● STIMULATION ACUPRESSURE POINT
● SEDATION ACUPRESSURE POINT
○ ELEMENTAL ACUPRESSURE POINT*
●-○- ALARM ACUPRESSURE POINT
-○- YU (ASSOCIATED) ACUPRESSURE POINT
● SUPERFICIAL ACUPRESSURE POINT
○ *SHICHEN MERIDIAN STRIKING POINT
◇ SHICHEN ZANFU 12 HOUR VITAL STRIKING POINT
□ GENERAL USE STRIKING POINTS

WRIST PULSE

LEFT	RIGHT
DEEP / SUPERFICIAL	DEEP / SUPERFICIAL
HT / LI	LU / LI
LV / GB	SP / ST
KD / BL	KD / PE - TW

The Meridians as Fields of Awareness

TCM uses Meridians in the same way one might contemplate a switchboard, only here, the meridian system is an **ecosystem**—not just **energy channels**, but **relational pathways through which the body organizes experience into meaning**:

- **Yin meridians stabilize** awareness, drawing Shen **inward** to deepen embodiment.
- **Yang meridians express** awareness, projecting Shen **outward** to engage with the world.
- **The Eight Extraordinary Vessels** provide **depth and continuity**, regulating Shen's ability to **process time, identity, and transformation.**

Meridians map the pathways between our Skin and the rest of our body. Every movement of Energy (Qi) through a meridian is also a **movement of Shen**—a **shift in perception, a change in relational attunement, a reorganization of embodied awareness**. Rather than viewing meridians as **fixed energy lines**, we can understand them as **living fields of experience**—a way to attune to the body through **motion, sensation, and perception**.

Each meridian relates to how we move through **three fundamental axes**: The Meridians as an Invitation to Sovereign Awareness. Shen are the entities in TCM that do the labor, and I define them many times, but at the end of the day, it's about how **you undersatand**. They are the Archetype of….

Yin and Yang are the foundation of all movement, all form, and all interaction. But **polarity alone is not enough**. The motion between opposites generates **energy**, but something must **guide and refine** that energy into awareness, intention, and coherence.

That something is **Shen (神).** In Taoist medicine, Shen is often translated as **"Spirit,"** but this is misleading if viewed through a **Western dualistic lens**. Shen is **not separate from the body**—it is the **awareness that emerges through the body's processes**:

- Through Qi (vital energy).
- Through blood and circulation.
- Through movement and breath.

If "Tion" defines something, then Shen describes it.

There is **Shen within the body**, and there is **cosmic Shen**—this system fully utilizes both, offering a **profoundly practical way to orient the mind toward embodied intelligence.**

The Five Phases of Traditional Chinese Medicine

Chinese medicine is based on a system called the 5 Phases, centering the elements of Wood, Fire, Earth, Metal, and Water. He is traditionally considered to have reigned around 2697–2597 BCE, though his existence is symbolic rather than historically confirmed. Huang Di is credited with numerous contributions to Chinese culture, science, medicine, and governance, often portrayed as a sage-king who guided humanity toward civilization.

Yin and Yang are the foundation of all movement, all form, and all interaction. But **polarity alone is not enough**. The motion between opposites generates **energy**, but something must **guide and refine** that energy into awareness, intention, and coherence.

That something is **Shen (神).**

In Taoist medicine, Shen is often translated as **"Spirit,"** but this is misleading if viewed through a **Western dualistic lens**. Shen is **not separate from the body**—it is the **awareness that emerges through the body's processes**:

- **Through Qi (vital energy).**
- **Through blood and circulation.**
- **Through movement and breath.**

If "Tion" defines something, then Shen describes it.

There is **Shen within the body**, and there is **cosmic Shen**—this system fully utilizes both, offering a **profoundly practical way to orient the mind toward embodied intelligence.**

Mapping the 5 Phases to the Human Body: Organ Pairings

I'm located in the US, where Acupuncture is a restricted practice, governed by Licensure. This creates clear scopes of practice, and the best way for me to stay in mine is for us to contemplate the Meridians through Shen. The main meridians represent parings of Yin and Yang organs:

Yin Organs (Zang): Full (Heart, Liver, Spleen, Lungs, Kidneys).

Yang Organs (Fu): Fill and empty cyclically (Small Intestine, Gallbladder, Stomach, Large Intestine, Bladder).

The following pages introduce you to the Shen by way of their Meridians. I've also included mappings to attributes like season, taste, and color, so you can personalize how you think about them. If you are more resonant with objects, shapes, or materials, please use them!

I also included flashcards for the Breathing Exercises, so you have them here as well as through the media you can access.

The Shen of the Five Yin Organs

Each organ has its own **resident Shen**, forming a **system of embodied awareness**:

- **Heart (Shen)** → Consciousness, clarity, perception.
- **Liver (Hun)** → Vision, movement, creative direction.
- **Spleen (Yi)** → Intellect, memory, grounded awareness.
- **Lungs (Po)** → Instinct, grief, embodied presence.
- **Kidneys (Zhi)** → Willpower, resilience, deep knowing.

This section invites you to:

- **Journal with Shen.**
- **Explore its resonances in Sound Healing & Somatics.**
- **Engage directly with these intelligences through breath and movement.**

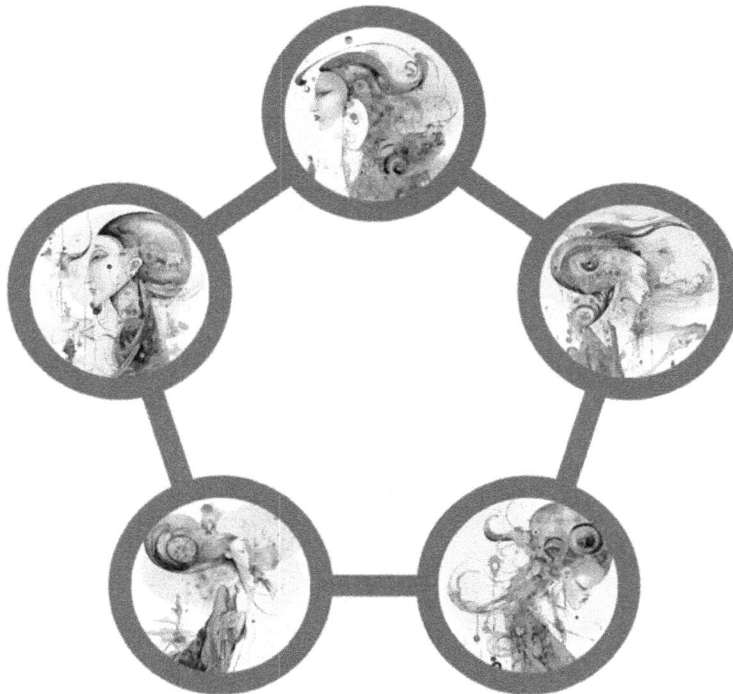

"Cheat Sheet" for the Shen and their Attributes

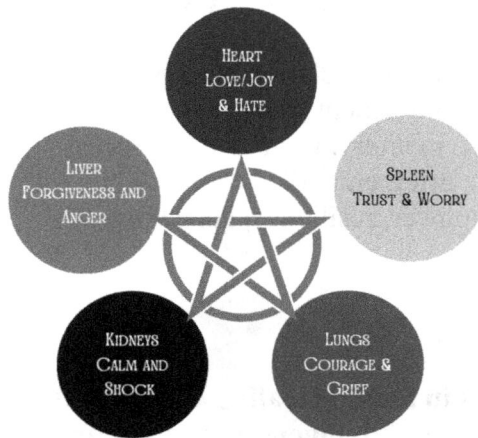

Katherine Zitterbart, MA IBOSP 617-543-9642 hello@kayteezee.com   KAYTEEZEE.COM

ORGAN>	Shen (神) (Heart)	Hun (魂) (Liver)	Po (魄) (Lungs)	Yi (意) (Spleen)	Zhi (志) (Kidneys -)
Element	Fire (火)	Wood (木)	Metal (金)	Earth (土)	Water (水)
Emotion	Joy (喜)	Anger (怒)	Grief (悲)	Worry (思)	Fear (恐)
Flavor	Bitter (苦)	Sour (酸)	Pungent (辛)	Sweet (甘)	Salty (咸)
Sense Organ	Tongue (舌)	Eyes (目)	Nose (鼻)	Mouth (口)	Ears (耳)
Sound	"Haaaaaa"	"Shhh"	"Ssss"	"Whooo"	"Choo"
Season	Summer (夏)	Spring (春)	Fall (秋)	Late Summer (长夏)	Winter (冬)
Color	Red (红)	Green (绿)	White (白)	Yellow (黄)	Blue/Black (蓝/黑)
Direction	South (南)	East (东)	West (西)	Center (中)	North (北)
Planet	Mars (火星)	Jupiter (木星)	Venus (金星)	Saturn (土星)	Mercury (水星)
Climate	Heat (热)	Wind (风)	Dryness (燥)	Dampness (湿)	Cold (寒)
Tissues	Blood vessels (脉)	Tendons (筋)	Skin (皮)	Muscles (肉)	Bones (骨)

(Rossi, 2007)

Live Practice: Meet the Shen

LIVE PRACTICE: MEET THE SHEN

HEART & SMALL INTESTINE - FIRE

The Heart is considered the emperor of all the organs in Traditional Chinese Medicine, governing not just the physical circulation of blood, but also the spiritual aspect of consciousness—what the ancients called the Shen or spirit. When the heart is balanced, joy flows easily, and life feels full of connection and warmth. The Small Intestine, meanwhile, helps to separate what is pure from what is impure, not just in food but in thought and emotion. It aids in discernment, allowing you to understand what is essential and let go of the rest.

TThe heart is linked to speech and communication through its connection to the tongue. Emotional disturbances, such as anxiety, joylessness, or insomnia, are directly related to the Heart Meridian. In TCM, the heart is referred to as the "emperor" of the body, controlling overall harmony and balance.

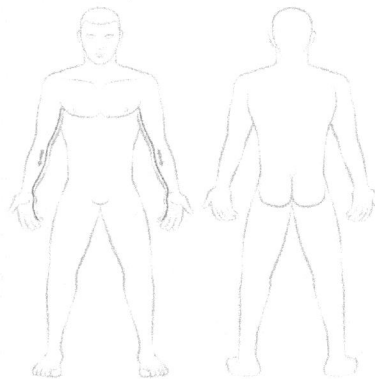

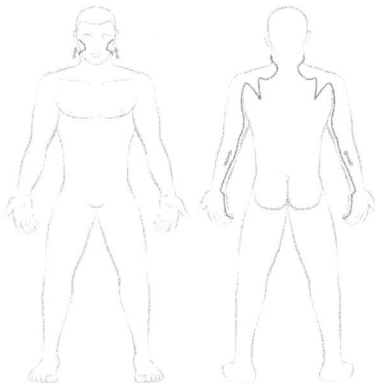

The Small Intestine Meridian is responsible for sorting and separating the pure from the impure, both in digestion and emotionally. It helps process and assimilate nutrients and experiences, providing clarity of thought and discernment. It is connected to the heart through their shared element (Fire), which is why emotional clarity and physical digestion are often linked. This meridian also influences the sense of direction in life.

SHEN: SPIRIT OF THE HEART

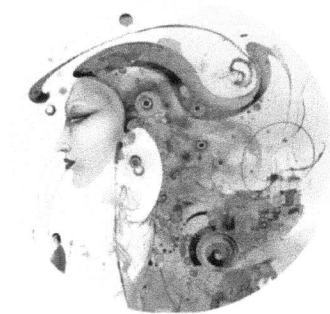

The Shen is the most central of the five spirits, often considered the consciousness or spirit of the person. It governs awareness, intelligence, mental clarity, and emotional expression. When Shen is balanced, one is calm, focused, and able to express love and compassion. It shines through the eyes, often referred to as the "light in the eyes."

Emotion: Joy (喜)
Healing Sound: "Haa" (like a sigh of relief)
Taste: Bitter (苦)
Season: Summer (夏)
Color: Red (红)
Planet: Mars (火星)
Direction: South (南)
Climate: Heat (热)
Sense Organ: Tongue (舌)
Tissues: Blood vessels (脉)
Virtue: Propriety, respect (礼)
Disharmony: Anxiety, insomnia, restlessness

In a Mirror

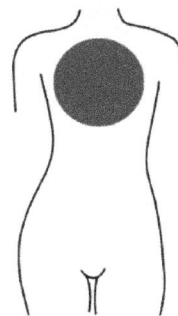

Katherine Zitterbart   617-543-9642   hello@kayteezee.com   kayteezee.com.   All Rights Reserved

The Heart and Shen (神): The Light of Consciousness

- **Organ:** Heart (Xin, 心)
- **Element:** Fire
- **Emotion:** Joy (Xi, 喜)
- **Shen's Psychoemotional Role:**
  The Heart houses **Shen**, the **primary spirit**, which governs **consciousness, awareness, mental clarity, emotions, and connection to the external world.** Shen is the light of awareness, responsible for **emotional regulation, relationships, and spiritual inspiration.**

Psychoemotional Aspects:

- **Healthy Shen:**
  - Mental clarity, calmness, and a strong connection to self and others.
  - Emotions, particularly **joy**, are experienced appropriately, without overexcitement or suppression.
  - A balanced Shen reflects in **stable moods**, the ability to remain present, and the capacity to regulate the nervous system.
  - The Heart-Shen oversees the **ventral vagal state**, enabling safe social engagement and emotional connection (parasympathetic dominance).
- **Disturbed Shen:**
  - Manifestations include **anxiety, insomnia, restlessness, and emotional dysregulation.**
  - When the Shen is disturbed, the nervous system oscillates between **hyperarousal** (sympathetic overdrive) and **dysregulated hypoarousal** (collapse or withdrawal).
  - Shen disturbance is also linked to **racing thoughts, palpitations, and difficulty concentrating.**
- **Heart-Shen and Nervous System Resonance:**
  - **Joy** (Xi, 喜), when balanced, supports **vagal tone** and fosters emotional resilience.
  - Excess joy or mania (hyperactive Shen) can lead to **nervous system dysregulation**, while deficient Shen may cause **apathy or disconnection.**

LIVER & GAL BLADDER - WOOD

The Liver and Gallbladder, under the influence of the Wood element, are the driving forces of growth, movement, and decision-making. The Liver is responsible for the smooth flow of Qi throughout the body. It detoxifies both physically and emotionally, processing not just waste but also anger, frustration, and irritability. When the Liver is blocked, these emotions can stagnate, leading to emotional outbursts or physical symptoms like headaches or menstrual irregularities.

The Liver Meridian is responsible for the smooth flow of Qi and blood throughout the body. It detoxifies the body and processes emotions, especially anger, frustration, and irritability. The liver stores blood and ensures the body's energy flows smoothly, preventing stagnation that can lead to physical and emotional blockages. It also governs the eyes and is associated with both physical vision and emotional clarity.

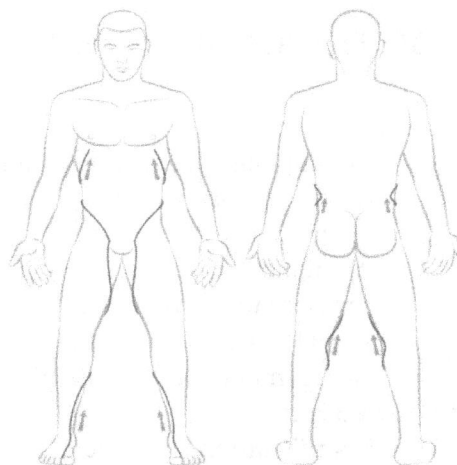

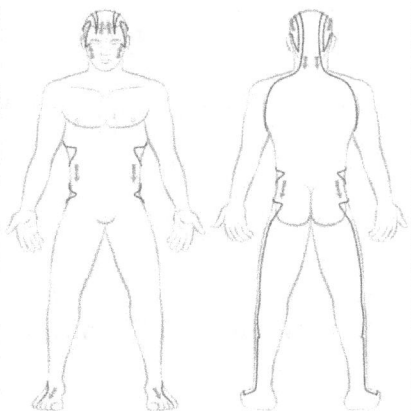

The Gallbladder Meridian controls decision-making, courage, and the ability to take action. It stores and secretes bile, aiding in the digestion of fats. Emotionally, the Gallbladder Meridian is linked to frustration, indecision, and suppressed anger. The sense organ associated with the gallbladder is the eyes, which governs vision, not just in terms of sight but also in the sense of "seeing" life's direction and having a clear vision.

Katherine Zitterbart   617-543-9642   hello@kayteezee.com   kayteezee.com.   All Rights Reserved

HUN - Spirit of the Liver - Wood

The Hun represents the ethereal or non-material aspect of the soul. It governs intuition, creativity, dreams, and long-term vision. The Hun is responsible for planning and decision-making, helping us navigate life's challenges. It leaves the body during sleep and returns upon waking, making it closely tied to imagination and spiritual growth.

Yin Organ: Liver (肝)
Shen: Hun (魂) – Ethereal soul
Emotion: Anger (怒)
Healing Sound: "Shh"
Taste: Sour (酸)
Season: Spring (春)
Color: Green (绿)
Planet: Jupiter (木星)
Direction: East (东)
Climate: Wind (风)
Sense Organ: Eyes (目)
Tissues: Tendons (筋)
Virtue: Kindness (仁)
Disharmony:

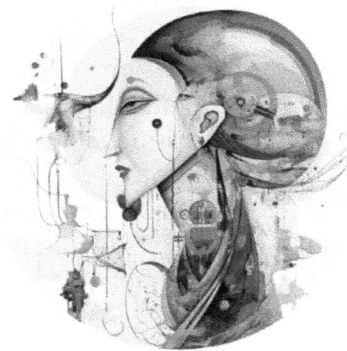

In a Mirror

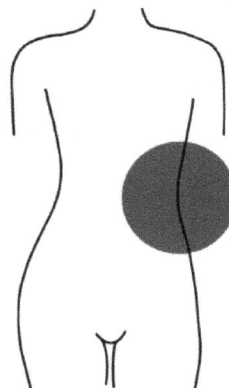

Katherine Zitterbart   617-543-9642   hello@kayteezee.com   kayteezee.com.   All Rights Reserved

The Liver and Hun (魂): The Ethereal Soul

- **Organ:** Liver (Gan, 肝)
- **Element:** Wood
- **Emotion:** Anger (Nu, 怒)
- **Hun's Psychoemotional Role:**
  The **Hun** governs **dreams, imagination, vision, and the capacity to plan for the future.** It is the **ethereal soul**, responsible for creative energy and forward momentum in life. Psychologically, Hun is tied to **decision-making, emotional expression, and ambition.**

Psychoemotional Aspects:

- **Healthy Hun:**
  - A vibrant Hun provides **clear vision, healthy assertiveness, and the ability to transform frustration into constructive action.**
  - The Liver-Hun supports **flexibility and adaptability**, key aspects of **emotional regulation** and maintaining **nervous system balance** during stress.
  - A regulated Hun allows the nervous system to move through sympathetic activation and into calm resolution, especially when overcoming challenges.
- **Disturbed Hun:**
  - **Anger** and frustration can stagnate the Liver energy, leading to emotional outbursts, irritability, or resentment.
  - Conversely, deficient Hun manifests as **indecision, hopelessness, or lack of vision.**
  - Chronic anger or stagnation overwhelms the sympathetic nervous system, keeping the body in a state of **fight-or-flight.**
- **Liver-Hun and Nervous System Resonance:**
  - The Hun helps the nervous system resolve frustration by transforming stagnation into **movement and flow.**
  - Liver Qi stagnation leads to **sympathetic overactivation** (e.g., tension, irritability), while Liver Qi that flows freely fosters **emotional resilience** and a balanced nervous system

Lungs & Large Intestine - Metal

The Lung and Large Intestine meridians, governed by the Metal element, represent structure, clarity, and the ability to let go. Metal is associated with grief—a heavy, dense emotion that can settle deep within the lungs, causing both physical and emotional blockages. But grief, when processed, makes space for something equally profound: courage. Courage is the energy of release, the act of trusting in the inhale and exhale, the flow of Qi moving smoothly through the lungs.

The Lung Meridian is the controller of Qi (vital energy) and respiration, governing the intake of air and the movement of Qi throughout the body. It opens to the nose, affecting the nasal passages, the skin, and body hair. In TCM, the lungs are also closely associated with the immune system, protecting the body from external pathogens. Grief and sadness are the primary emotions that affect the lungs.

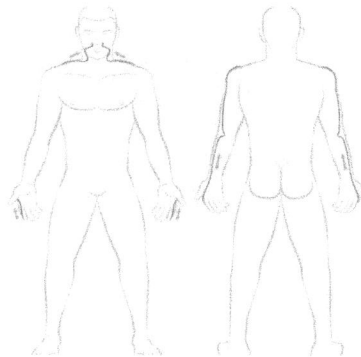

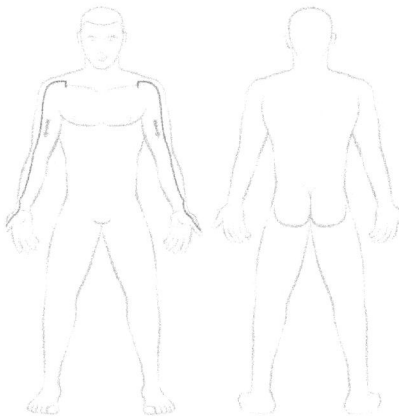

The Large Intestine Meridian is responsible for the elimination of waste and toxins from the body. It plays a vital role in both digestion and the body's ability to let go of what is no longer needed—both physically and emotionally. As it is paired with the Lung Meridian, it is connected to respiration and is affected by the same emotional issues related to grief and attachment. In TCM, a blocked Large Intestine Meridian can lead to constipation, skin problems, and an inability to release emotional baggage.

PO - Spirit of the Lungs/Metal

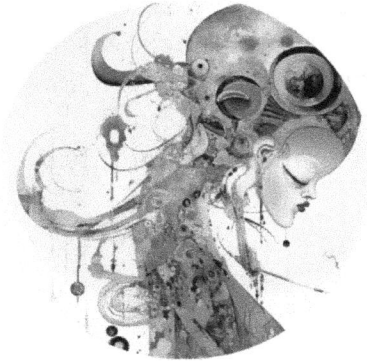

The Po is the corporeal, physical soul, linked to bodily sensations and survival instincts. It is responsible for our connection to the physical world and governs the body's automatic processes, such as breathing. The Po is deeply connected to the present moment and bodily experiences, and it dissipates upon death. Imbalances in Po can manifest as grief or difficulty in letting go.

Emotion: Grief (悲)
Healing Sound: "Sss" (like a hissing sound)
Taste: Pungent (辛)
Season: Autumn (秋)
Color: White (白)
Planet: Venus (金星)
Direction: West (西)
Climate: Dryness (燥)
Sense Organ: Nose (鼻)
Tissues: Skin (皮)
Virtue: Righteousness (义)
Disharmony: Sadness, difficulty letting go

Your Back

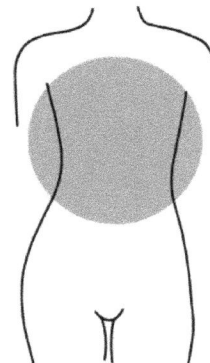

Katherine Zitterbart   617-543-9642   hello@kayteezee.com   kayteezee.com.   All Rights Reserved

The Lungs and Po (魄): The Corporeal Soul

- **Organ:** Lungs (Fei, 肺)
- **Element:** Metal
- **Emotion:** Grief (Bei, 悲)
- **Po's Psychoemotional Role:**
  The **Po** is the **corporeal soul**, responsible for physical sensations, survival instincts, and the body's connection to the material world. It governs the **somatic experience of emotion**, as well as the ability to let go and move through grief.

Psychoemotional Aspects:

- **Healthy Po:**
  - A strong Po enables the ability to **process loss** and move through emotional transitions with acceptance and grace.
  - It allows for full embodiment and awareness of physical sensations, fostering a **somatic connection** that supports **nervous system regulation.**
  - Healthy Po supports the parasympathetic state, promoting deep breathing and calming of the nervous system.
- **Disturbed Po:**
  - **Unresolved grief** can overwhelm the Po, leading to **chronic sadness, detachment, or a sense of being stuck in the past.**
  - This may manifest as **difficulty letting go** of experiences, emotional numbness, or excessive clinging to physical attachments.
  - The nervous system may remain in a **dysregulated parasympathetic state** (e.g., freeze or collapse) or become hyperactive due to unresolved emotional pain.
- **Lungs-Po and Nervous System Resonance:**
  - Deep, rhythmic breathing (a Lung function) is essential for **vagus nerve activation** and regulating the nervous system.
  - Grief, when acknowledged and processed, allows the Po to restore a sense of **groundedness and physical safety.**

STOMACH & SPLEEN - EARTH

Grounded in the Earth element, the Stomach and Spleen meridians are the cornerstones of digestion—not just of food, but of thoughts, emotions, and life experiences. Earth is stable, nurturing, and supportive, embodying the qualities of trust and worry. When the Earth element is balanced, you feel nourished and secure, both in your body and in your thoughts. But when imbalance strikes, worry takes root, like a storm cloud hovering over the mind, disrupting the digestive process of both body and soul.

The Spleen Meridian is essential for digestion and the production of Qi and blood, as well as the transport and transformation of nutrients. It governs the muscles, the flesh, and is deeply involved in mental clarity, focus, and concentration. In TCM, the spleen is the central organ of nourishment, and its health is tied to a person's capacity for sustained mental effort. Worry, overthinking, and obsessive behavior are emotions that disturb the spleen. Dry lips and a lack of appetite are physical signs of imbalances.

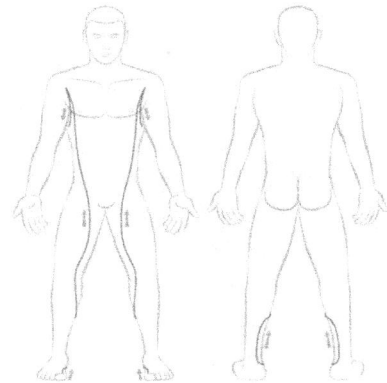

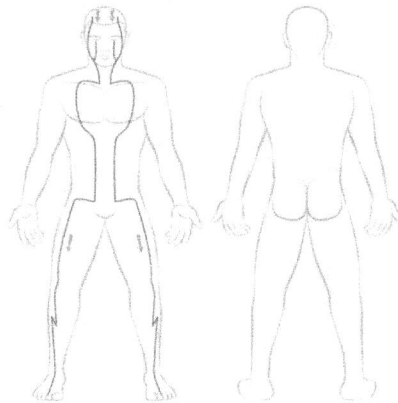

The Stomach Meridian governs the intake, digestion, and processing of food, thoughts, and emotions. It is considered one of the most important meridians in TCM due to its role in generating Qi and blood. When balanced, the stomach is strong and able to process nourishment, but when out of balance, it can lead to digestive disturbances, worry, and overthinking. The Stomach Meridian is associated with the mouth and sense of taste, which is why digestive problems often affect appetite and taste.

YI: Spirit of the Spleen / Earth

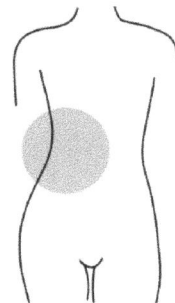

The Yi refers to the intellect and is responsible for analytical thinking, focus, and memory. It represents the ability to study, concentrate, and form intentions. A strong Yi allows one to make sound decisions, while an imbalanced Yi may result in overthinking, worry, or obsessive thoughts.

Emotion: Worry (忧)
Healing Sound: "Hoo" (like blowing softly)
Taste: Sweet (甜)
Season: Late Summer (长夏)
Color: Yellow (黄)
Planet: Saturn (土星)
Direction: Center (中)
Climate: Dampness (湿)
Sense Organ: Mouth (口)
Tissues: Muscles (肉)
Virtue: Integrity (信)
Disharmony: Overthinking, obsession, lack of focus

In a Mirror

Katherine Zitterbart   617-543-9642   hello@kayteezee.com   kayteezee.com. All Rights Reserved

The Spleen and Yi (意): The Intellect

- **Organ:** Spleen (Pi, 脾)
- **Element:** Earth
- **Emotion:** Worry (Si, 思)
- **Yi's Psychoemotional Role:**
  The **Yi** governs **intellect, thought, and concentration**, as well as the ability to process and integrate experiences. It supports **mental focus and the formation of intention**, bridging thought and action.

Psychoemotional Aspects:

- **Healthy Yi:**
  - A balanced Yi fosters **clarity of thought**, mental resilience, and the ability to **reflect without overthinking.**
  - Emotional regulation relies on the Spleen's ability to process information and experiences, ensuring the mind remains **centered and grounded.**
- **Disturbed Yi:**
  - Excessive worry, rumination, or overthinking can weaken the Yi, leading to **mental fatigue, confusion, and difficulty focusing.**
  - Chronic worry reflects **Spleen Qi deficiency**, which can dysregulate the nervous system by keeping it in a heightened state of **mental activity** without resolution.
  - Nervous system dysregulation may manifest as **sympathetic overdrive**, with looping thoughts and difficulty calming the mind.
- **Spleen-Yi and Nervous System Resonance:**
  - The Yi helps the nervous system return to a **regulated parasympathetic state** by resolving mental clutter and worry.
  - Practices like grounding and mindfulness directly support the Yi, allowing the Spleen to digest mental and emotional experiences.

KIDNEYS & BLADDER - WATER

The Kidneys hold the body's most vital essence, or Jing, and are the source of life force. They govern growth, reproduction, and longevity. Emotionally, the Kidneys are tied to fear and courage—the primal forces of survival. Chronic fear can deplete the Kidneys, leading to exhaustion, while courage strengthens them, providing deep reservoirs of energy and vitality.

The Kidney Meridian is one of the most important in TCM as it stores the body's vital essence, known as "Jing." The kidneys are considered the source of life force, governing reproduction, growth, aging, and longevity. Emotionally, the Kidney Meridian is related to fear and survival instincts. Chronic fear and exhaustion can deplete kidney energy, leading to fatigue, low back pain, and issues related to fertility or bone health. In TCM, the ears are the sense organ governed by the kidneys, and hearing problems can indicate a kidney imbalance.

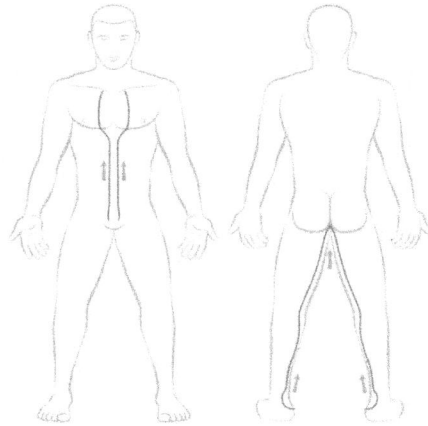

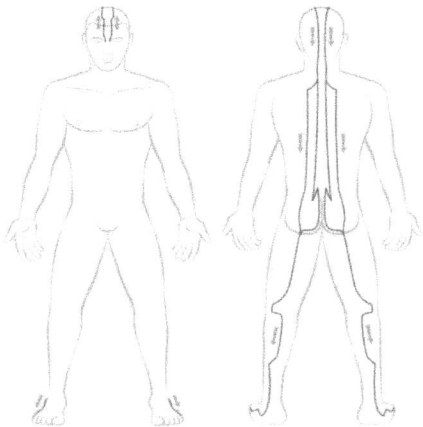

The Bladder Meridian is the longest meridian in the body, running from the head down to the toes, and it governs the excretion of fluids and waste. In TCM, it is closely linked to the nervous system and emotional responses, especially fear and anxiety. The bladder stores and excretes fluids, but it also holds emotional tension, particularly along the spine, where the Bladder Meridian runs. Hearing issues can sometimes be related to Bladder Meridian imbalances.

Zhi ꞉ Spirit of the Kidneys

The Zhi represents willpower, drive, and determination. It governs our ambition, perseverance, and ability to follow through with goals. A strong Zhi gives one the strength to face fear and overcome obstacles, while a weak Zhi may lead to fearfulness, low motivation, or a sense of helplessness.

Emotion: Fear (恐)
Healing Sound: "Choo" (like exhaling cool air)
Taste: Salty (咸)
Season: Winter (冬)
Color: Black (黑)
Planet: Mercury (水星)
Direction: North (北)
Climate: Cold (寒)
Sense Organ: Ears (耳)
Tissues: Bones (骨)
Virtue: Wisdom (智)
Disharmony: Fearfulness, low motivation, fatigue

Your Back

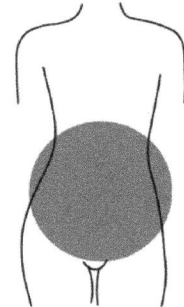

Katherine Zitterbart   617-543-9642   hello@kayteezee.com   kayteezee.com.   All Rights Reserved

The Kidneys and Zhi (志): The Willpower

- **Organ:** Kidneys (Shen, 肾)
- **Element:** Water
- **Emotion:** Fear (Kong, 恐)
- **Zhi's Psychoemotional Role:**
  The **Zhi** governs **willpower, determination, and resilience.** It represents our capacity to endure challenges and stay aligned with our life purpose. The Zhi reflects the depth of one's **emotional reserves** and ability to face fears with courage.

Psychoemotional Aspects:

- **Healthy Zhi:**
  - A strong Zhi manifests as **resilience, courage, and the ability to act in the face of uncertainty.**
  - The Kidneys house our **ancestral energy (Jing)**, providing the foundation for survival instincts and nervous system stability.
- **Disturbed Zhi:**
  - Imbalanced Zhi results in **fear, insecurity, or a sense of paralysis.**
  - Chronic fear weakens the Kidneys, leading to **sympathetic overactivation** and difficulty calming the body.
  - Conversely, deficient Kidney Zhi leads to **collapse** or a sense of hopelessness (dysregulated parasympathetic state).
- **Kidneys-Zhi and Nervous System Resonance:**
  - The Zhi regulates how we respond to stress and fear, directly influencing the **HPA axis** (hypothalamus-pituitary-adrenal system).
  - A resilient Zhi supports **nervous system recovery** after stress, while weak Zhi can leave the system in chronic fight-or-flight.

The Governing Vessel   **The Conception Vessel**

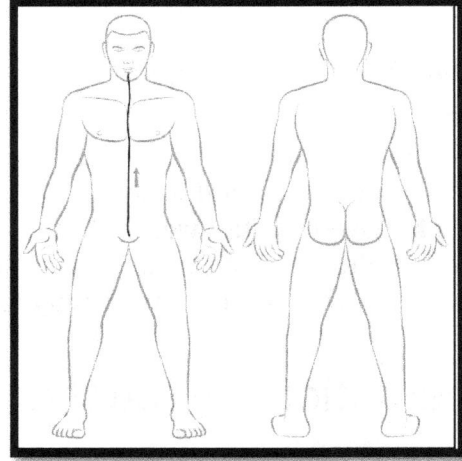

Sea of Yang   Sea of Yin

Bridging the Meridians, Governing & Conception Vessels → Neijing Tu & Neidan

These two meridians operate as a bridge between the Macrocosm and the Microcosm, and they align to our Cerebrospinal Fluid. They are personified by two of the 8 Immortals, whom you will meet soon.

First, I want to guide you to the main map of Neidan, so you can meet more Shen – and if you want to skip ahead, please do so.

The **Governing Vessel (Du Mai)** and **Conception Vessel (Ren Mai)** are the **primary regulators of structure and flow**, shaping how **energy moves, organizes, and transforms** within us.

◆ **The Conception Vessel (Ren Mai) gathers, nourishes, and integrates Yin energy.**
◆ **The Governing Vessel (Du Mai) guides, activates, and expresses Yang energy.**
◆ **Together, they create the first polarity of life—flowing up the spine and down the front of the body, forming a circuit of dynamic exchange.**

But the **Neijing Tu** takes us deeper. It does not just trace **Qi through these pathways**—it reveals **how these currents shape perception, transformation, and consciousness itself.**

Following are flashcards for the organ resonance. There are lessons and more in the Media you can access via the QR Codes .

PRACTICE: Organ Yoga with the Shen

To practice with your own Shen, all you need to do is direct your attention inward, thusly:

GRAVITY | SENSE OF BUM

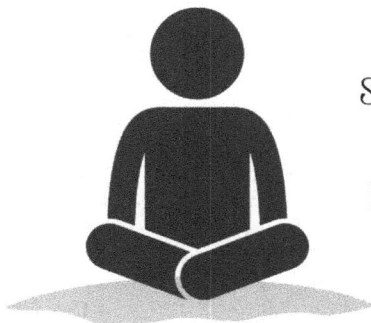

SENSE OF BUM HELPS
US REMEMBER WE
EXIST AND ARE PART
OF THE EQUATION

Take a couple breaths in through your nose and out
of your mouth. Settle ONTO the surface. Is it hard?
are you sitting? Can you feel the places where you
and There connect?
THAT IS YOUR SENSE OF BUM
That's it – find gravity and Notice. This is challenging
for some humans, so be compassionate towards Self.

Katherine Zitterbart, MA IBOSP 617-543-9642 hello@kayteezee.com   KAYTEEZEE.COM

THE HEALING SMILE

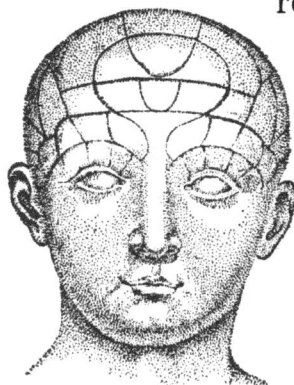

You can practice this with your eyes open while
reading this. In the future, you can practice with
eyes open or closed. If open - cast your gaze
towards something analog

Gently rest the tip of your tongue on the
ridge behind your upper teeth, allowing
the rest to relax

Signal "Smile" with your face - either
literally or on the inside. While you connect
with the smile, imagine you're smiling
towards your SOMA - your literal body

Smile to your organ, Breath In the Good – Let Go the Bad – Take 3-5 rounds per Organ

LUNGS - 1ST SOUND
COURAGE & GRIEF
SSSSSSSSSS

KIDNEYS - 2ND SOUND
SHOCK & CALM
CHOOOOOO

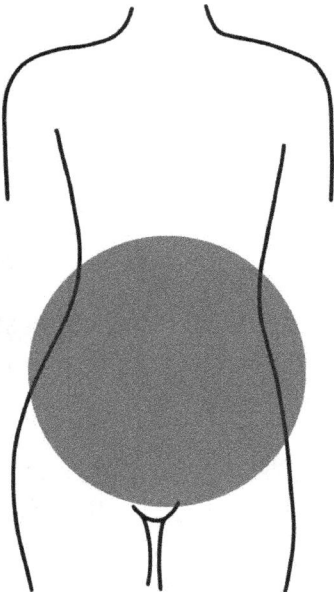

LIVER 3RD SOUND
ANGER & FORGIVENESS
SHHHHHHHHHH

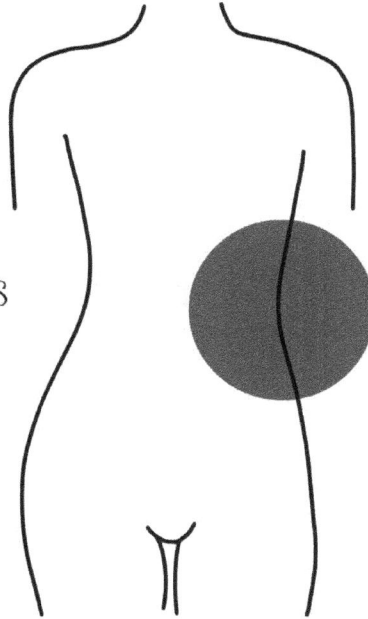

HEART 4TH SOUND
LOVE & HATE
HAAAAAAAAAA

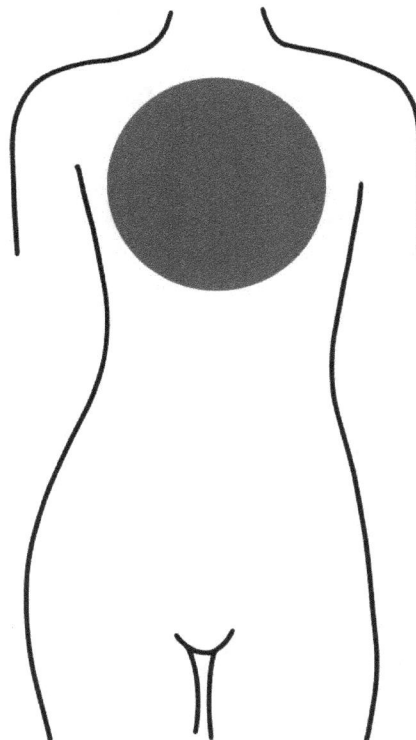

SPLEEN 5TH SOUND
TRUST & WORRY
WHOOOOOOO

Pericardium - Homeostasis
HEEEEEEEEEEE

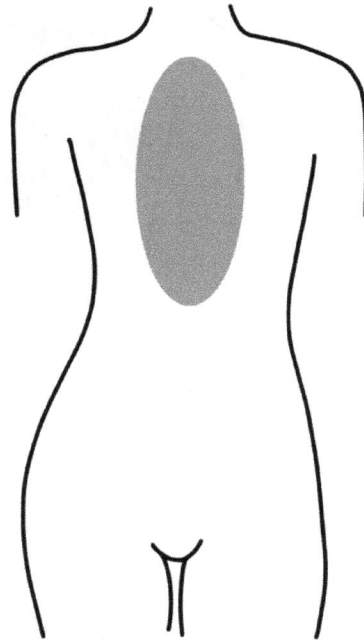

6th Sound

Charting the Lived Experience with the Neijing Tu

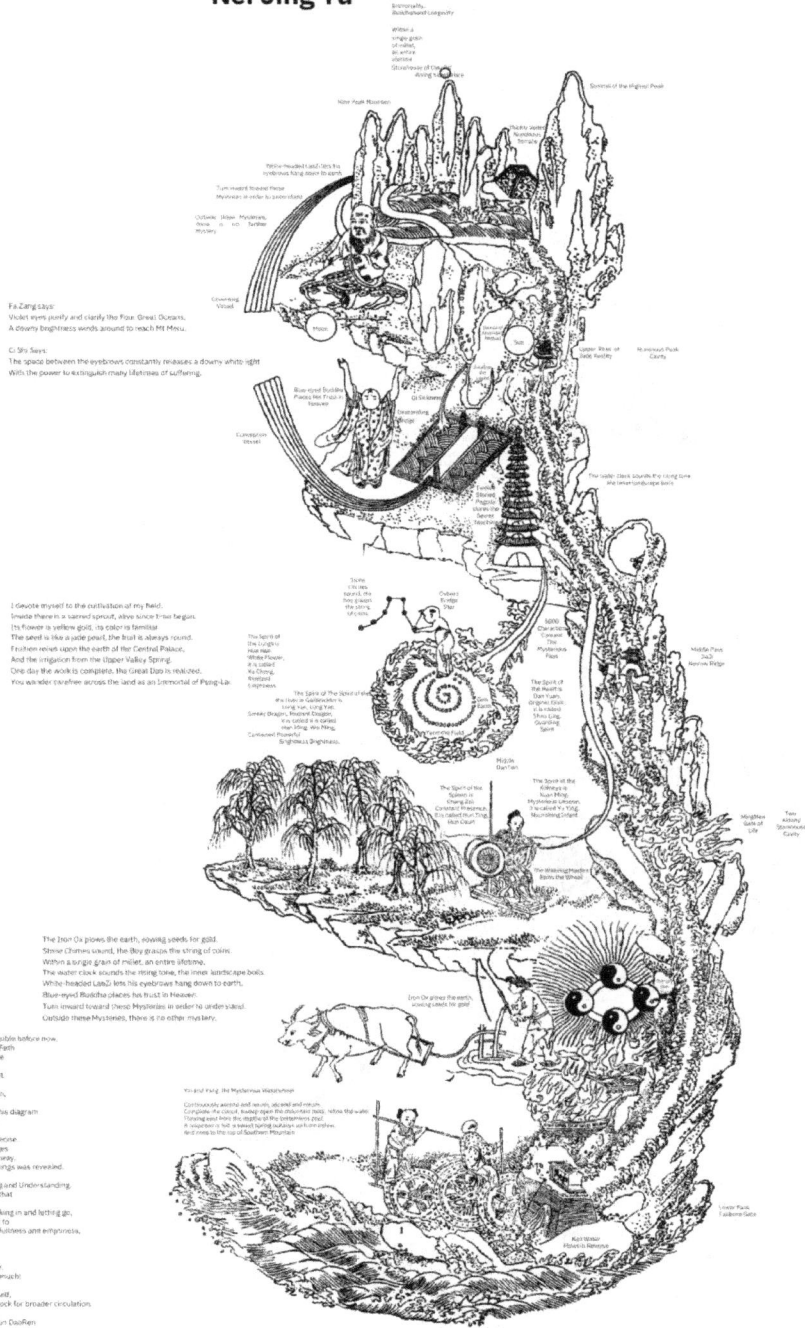

The Diagram of the Inner Realm
內經圖
Nei Jing Tu

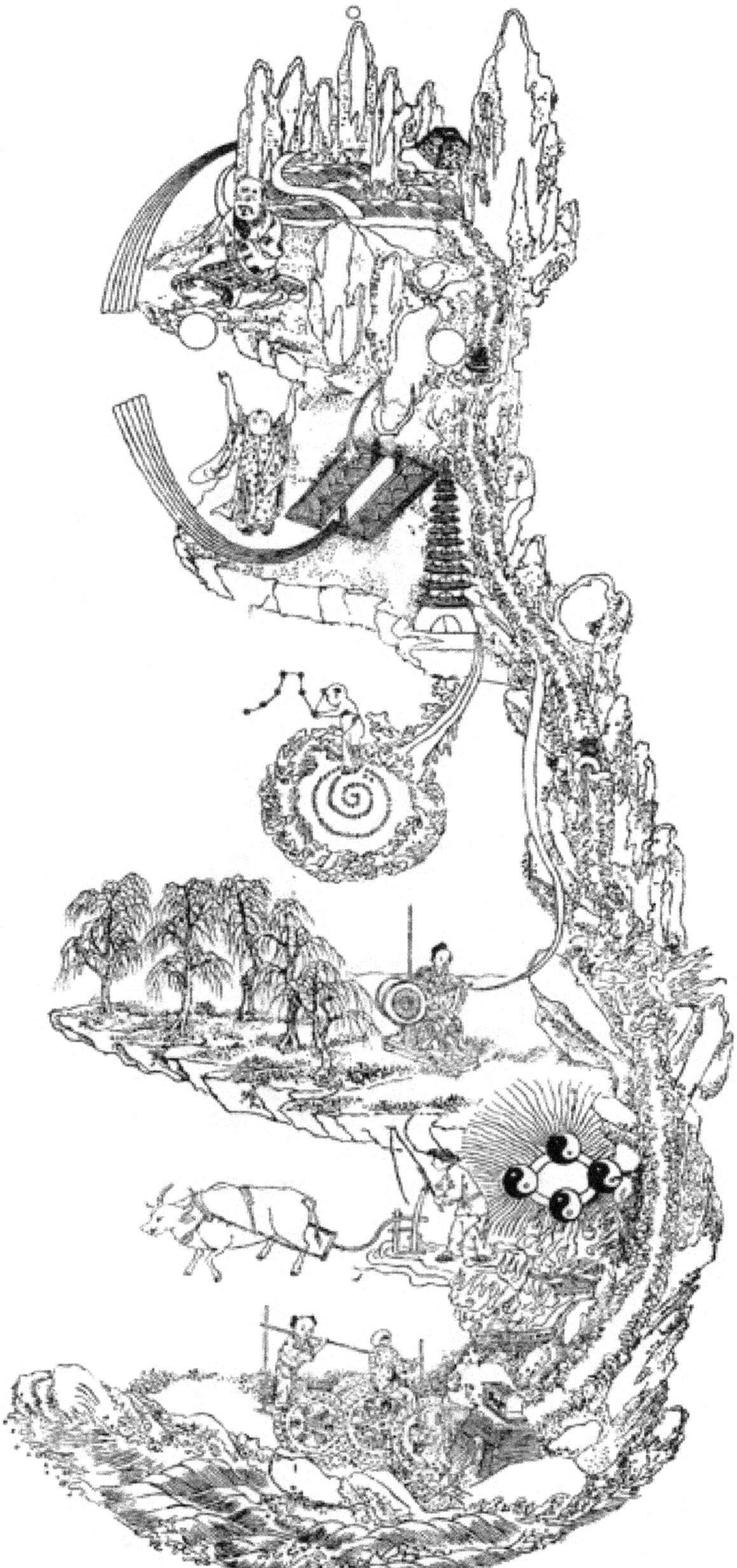

The Neijing Tu (knee-jing too) (內經圖) I a **map of embodied experience**, a way to sense the **flow of energy, perception, and movement within the body**. It is used in Acupuncture as well as Neidan – Inner Alchemy. From a Neidan Perspective, this chart provides a dynamic and accurate mapping of the stages of development we, as practitioners, engage in. Unlike modern anatomical charts, which focus on **fixed structures** (muscles, bones, and organs), the Neijing Tu depicts the **human form as a landscape**—with rivers, mountains, pathways, and celestial bodies.

The Neijing Tu is sometimes translated as **The Inner Warp**. When we contemplate it form that perspective, it becomes the fabric upon and through which the patterns of life emerge. This is the Matrix of Human, and as an interface, it is quite possibly the most brilliant map I have ever seen. As the

Why Does the Neijing Tu Matter?

1. **It Bridges Ancient Wisdom and Sensory Experience.**
   o Western anatomy charts show where things **are**—the Neijing Tu shows how they **move**.
   o It emphasizes **flow, resonance, and adaptability** over mechanical function.
   o Instead of dissecting the body, it invites us to **feel** it.
2. **It Maps the Journey of Shen, Not Just Qi.**
   o Meridians describe the flow of **Qi (vital energy)**, but the Neijing Tu charts the entire **process of perception and consciousness (Shen)**.
   o It includes the **Three Dantian (lower, middle, upper)**, linking **body, breath, and awareness**.
   o It integrates **nervous system function** with **energetic transformation**.
3. **It Reveals the Extraordinary Vessels—Pathways of Inheritance & Perception.**
   o Unlike the standard **12 meridians**, the Neijing Tu illuminates **the 8 Extraordinary Vessels**, which govern **ancestral memory, sensory perception, and deep nervous system regulation**.
   o These vessels act like **hidden rivers**, shaping how we experience time, emotion, and embodiment.
4. **It Helps Us See the Body as an Ecosystem, Not a Machine.**
   o Instead of **veins and nerves**, it shows **rivers and mountains**.
   o Instead of **muscles and bones**, it depicts **temples and celestial bodies**.
   o This shift in perception helps us experience the body as a **living, interconnected landscape**.

Video Tour of the Inner Realm: Neijing Tour

How to Read the Neijing Tu - 3 Energy Centers

The Neijing Tu illustrates three Energy Centers, called Dantian (dawn – TEE-en). The **Dantian (** 丹田**)** are not abstract concepts but tangible **places within**—each serving as a **palace** or **earth**, where we can settle, land, and attune to embodied experience. These centers are the foundation of **Neidan** (內丹), or Taoist Inner Alchemy, which teaches that transformation is only possible when there is **a stable center**. Without an earth to stand on, how can we walk the path?

In Taoist practice, **the success of our inner alchemy depends on the stability of the Earth at the central palace** (Middle Dantian). This is what allows us to move into the **literal** middle path—the Middle Way. When this balance is cultivated, **confusion dissolves**, and we find ourselves able to experience inner transformation **without force, without tension**.

This is also what makes the **Neijing Tu and Neidan practices inherently peaceful** and aligned with **trauma-informed principles**. By focusing on **grounding and integration** rather than control, these practices allow for **diverse experiences**—rather than a singular "correct" way of being.

Neuroaffective Brain – Neijing Tu

Due to it representing 1 Fertile Female, Neuroaffective Somatics interprets the Neijing Tu as "brain". These mappings are new and based on Jing Chi Shen, and the 3 Planes of the Brain.

- In modern neuroscience, the **Corpus Callosum** is the bridge that **integrates left and right brain function**—balancing rational thought with intuition, structure with fluidity.
- The Neijing Tu **mirrors this function**, showing how **resonance moves between different states of awareness**.
- The **12 Cranial Nerves**—which regulate sensory perception, facial expression, breath, and vagal tone—can be mapped onto the Neijing Tu's pathways of **Qi and Shen**.

This perspective **connects ancient embodiment wisdom with modern neurophysiology**, allowing us to see the Neijing Tu as both **a historical artifact and a living practice**.

The Neijing Tu is not just a **map of the body**—it is an invitation to experience yourself as a **dynamic, living landscape**.

The following section will break down the Neijing Tu **into layers**, allowing you to experience its fractal nature **firsthand**.

The Three Dantian and the Three Energies

If you recall, earlier I shared that there are three virtues in Taoism: Compassion, Moderation, and Humility. These virtues align to 3 energy centers we contemplate in Neidan, called Dantian (dawn-tee-in). The literal translation is Cauldron, such that we are contemplating the body has **having** space. The Dantian are locations where we "do" the alchemy, and just like Shen, they are automagic. Aligned to the Belly, the Heart, and the Head, they represent Earth, Humanity, and Heaven respectively.

Each of the **three Dantian** aligns with one of the **three primary types of energy in Taoist thought** (Chia, 1993): The following Pages guide you into these centers specifically and in ways that will help you apply the concepts to any framework you're already in.

1. **Lower Dantian (Xia Dantian - 下丹田) → Jing (精)**
   - The root, the base, the physical essence
   - Located below the navel, this center **grounds and stabilizes**
   - Associated with **ancestral energy, vitality, reproduction, and longevity**
   - Without **Jing**, we burn out, deplete, or feel unmoored from the body
2. **Middle Dantian (Zhong Dantian - 中丹田) → Qi (氣)**
   - The breath, the heart, the movement of life force
   - Located at the heart center, this is where **emotions, rhythm, and connection to others are cultivated**
   - It is the **Earth of the body**, where energy circulates and harmonizes
   - Without **Qi**, we feel disconnection, imbalance, or emotional instability
3. **Upper Dantian (Shang Dantian - 上丹田) → Shen (神)**
   - The mind, the spirit, perception and consciousness
   - Located in the forehead (third eye region), this is where **awareness and insight reside**
   - The **bridge to the ineffable**, where perception expands
   - Without **Shen**, we experience **mental restlessness, lack of clarity, or spiritual confusion**

Includes Neijing Tu Charts

FREE CHARTS AND BOOKLETS

Lower Dantian (Xia Dantian / Lower Palace) - Jing

- **Location**: The Lower Dantian is located in the abdomen, about three finger-widths below the navel. It is often described as the foundation of the human energy system.
- **Associated Energy: Jing (Essence)**: Jing is the densest and most foundational form of energy, closely linked to physical health, vitality, and longevity. It is considered the "seed" or "root" energy, fundamental for all life processes.
- **Role in Alchemical Practice**: The Lower Dantian is where Jing is stored, transformed, and conserved. In internal alchemy, cultivating the Lower Dantian strengthens the body's foundation, enhances physical resilience, and conserves energy that can later be refined into Chi and Shen. Practices focused on the Lower Dantian include qigong and breathing exercises aimed at building physical strength, grounding, and endurance.
- **Earth as Stability**: The Lower Dantian aligns with the grounding qualities of Earth, providing stability and a sense of rootedness. This center anchors the practitioner to their physical presence and cultivates an inner sense of stability, preparing the energy to be raised to higher planes.

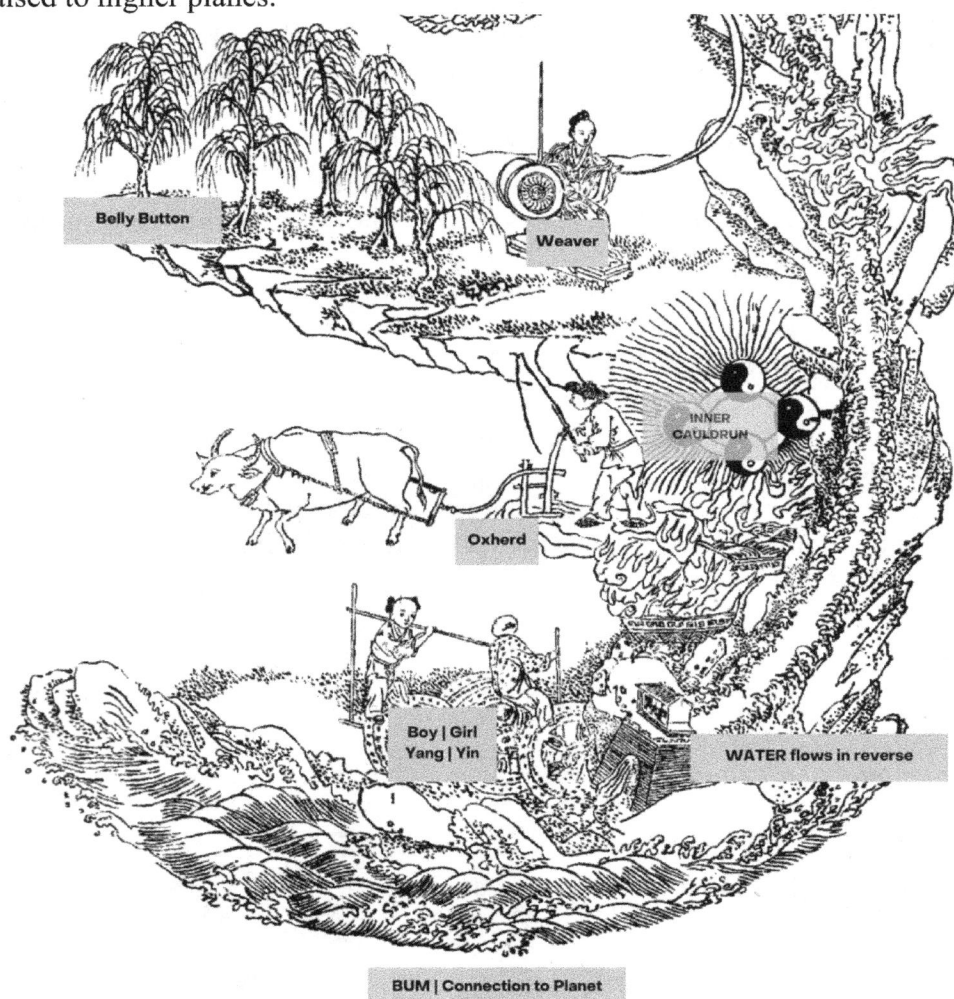

Middle Dantian (Zhong Dantian / Central Palace) - Chi

- **Location**: The Middle Dantian is located in the center of the chest, at the level of the heart. This area is associated with emotional balance and interpersonal connection.
- **Associated Energy: Chi (Life Force)**: Chi is the vital energy that circulates throughout the body, facilitating movement, breath, and the sustenance of life. It is often equated with the body's bioelectric energy and is essential for maintaining overall health and vitality.
- **Role in Alchemical Practice**: The Middle Dantian is the seat of Chi, and cultivating it allows practitioners to balance emotions, enhance empathy, and refine interpersonal awareness. This center transforms Jing into Chi, allowing physical energy to become more fluid and accessible. Practices focused on the Middle Dantian include heart-centered meditations, breathwork, and techniques aimed at emotional regulation and increasing compassion.
- **Earth as Heart Harmony**: In the context of internal alchemy, the Middle Dantian represents the Earth element's quality of harmony within oneself and with others. This center serves as the bridge between the physical and spiritual realms, balancing the denser energy of Jing with the lighter, more active energy of Shen.

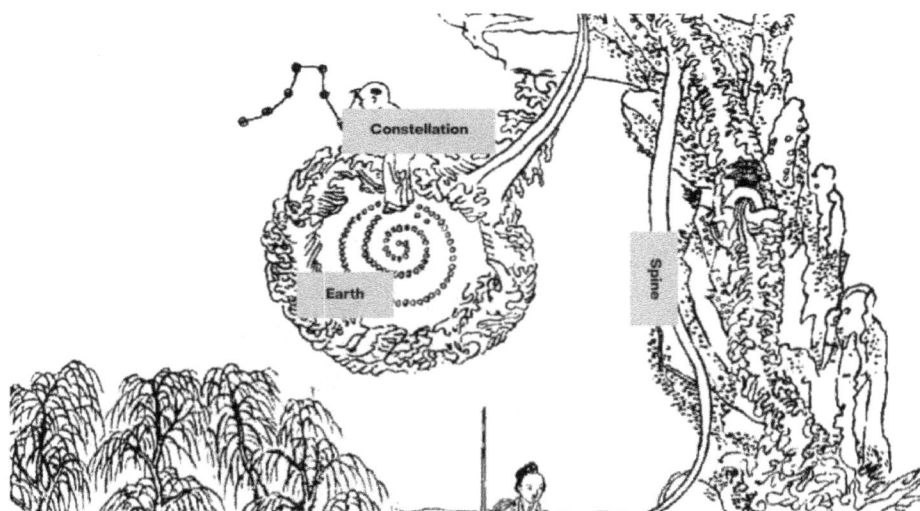

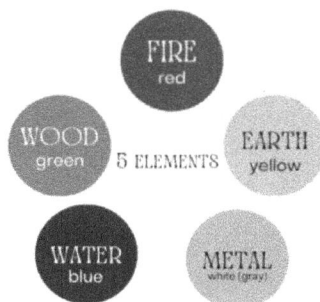

This Map places Emotional Alchemy in the Heart, illustrating the metaphoric placement of the Window of Tolerance

Upper Dantian (Shang Dantian / Crystal Palace) - Shen

- **Location**: The Upper Dantian is located in the center of the forehead, often referred to as the "Third Eye" area. It is associated with higher consciousness, intuition, and spiritual insight.
- **Associated Energy: Shen (Spirit)**: Shen represents the most refined and subtle form of energy, often equated with consciousness, spirit, or awareness. Shen is considered the seat of consciousness, and its cultivation leads to wisdom, clarity, and spiritual connection.
- **Shen as your Spirit**: Every sentient being has a Shen of Self/Soma – the whole spirit.
- **Role in Alchemical Practice**: The Upper Dantian is the center of Shen, and cultivating it allows practitioners to expand awareness, connect with spiritual realms, and gain insight into the nature of reality. This center transforms Chi into Shen, enabling practitioners to elevate their perception and experience a sense of unity with the Tao. Practices focused on the Upper Dantian include meditation, visualization, and techniques that develop intuitive insight and higher consciousness.
- **Earth as Elevated Consciousness**: The Upper Dantian embodies the transcendent qualities of Earth, where stability is found not through physical grounding but through the anchoring of consciousness. This center allows practitioners to "ground" their awareness in a higher reality, providing stability in the realm of thought, intuition, and spirit.

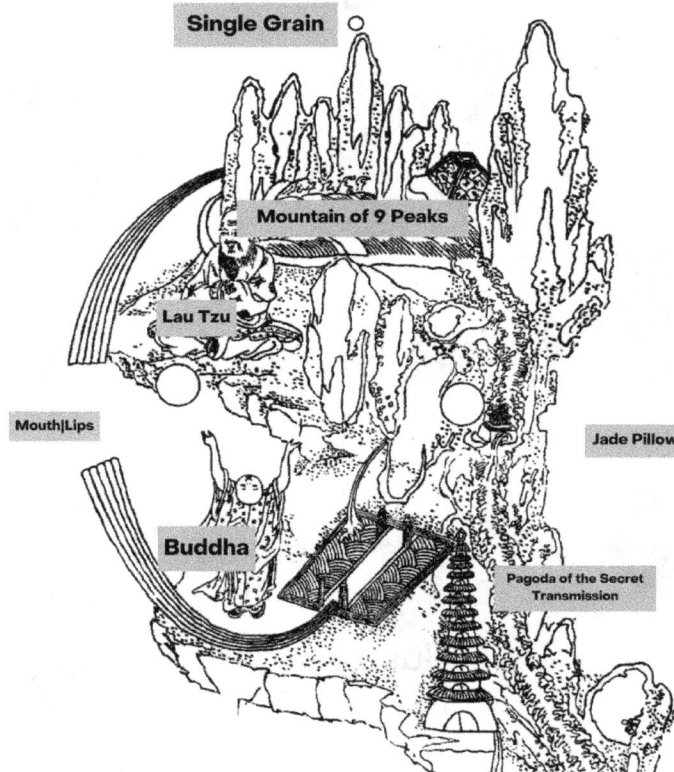

Katherine Zitterbart, MA IBOSP 617-543-9642 hello@kayteezee.com   KAYTEEZEE.COM

Unlike modern anatomical drawings that separate parts into **mechanical components**, the Neijing Tu sees the body as a **landscape of flowing energy, intelligence, and symbiosis.** It does not divide humans from nature but instead **situates us within it**—as part of the same forces that shape rivers, mountains, and winds.

We are **animals, bipedal great apes of the genus Homo, embedded in the same living systems as all creatures.** The Neijing Tu reminds us of this by depicting the human form **not as a mechanical body, but as a landscape of process and relationship.**

Just as Western biology classifies living things into **Kingdom, Phylum, Class, Order, Family, Genus, and Species**, the Neijing Tu **depicts levels of experience, development, and Shen through recognizable figures.**

These characters are **not separate beings**—they represent **processes unfolding in every human body. They are Shen.** Each figure in the Neijing Tu corresponds not only to **energetic processes** but to our **deep biological nature.**

The Shen of the Neijing Tu: A Bottom-Up Introduction

Exploring Shen through Biological Classification, Taoist Alchemy, and Somatic Experience

The Neijing Tu offers a **non-anatomical** but deeply **embodied** map of the human experience. Rather than a literal depiction of organs or systems, it presents a **symbolic topography** of consciousness, energy, and somatic intelligence.

By aligning its figures with **biological classification**, we shift from the hierarchical view of "human exceptionalism" toward an integrated **animal experience**. We are not "separate from nature" but part of the vast continuum of life. This approach allows us to explore the **layers of Shen**—from the grounding of our species to the expansiveness of our soul.

CORPUS CALLOSUM & THE NEIJING TU FROM

Corpus Callosum Audio Lesson

Engage with the Shen of the Neijing Tu – Data & ContemplaShens

Having explored the **Neijing Tu (內經圖)** and the **Dantian system**, we now turn to a new layer of contemplation: how these **Shen (spirit-intelligences)** relate to both **biological evolution and the nervous system.**

The **Neijing Tu is not just a metaphorical map—it is a dynamic model of embodied perception.** It does not depict the brain as an object, but rather as an **interactive continuum of movement, awareness, and refinement.**

In this model, each figure in the **Neijing Tu corresponds to a neurological function**, revealing how **Daoist alchemy engages with the nervous system, the sensorimotor experience, and the progressive refinement of perception.**

This mapping follows a clear sequence:

- **We begin with the foundation of Yin and Yang, where raw sensory and motor coordination take form.**
- **From there, each stage reflects an increasingly refined interaction between structure, sensation, and awareness.**
- **At the highest levels, perception is no longer reactive but fluid, integrated, and responsive.**

Resonance as the Core of Nervous System Function

Resonance in this context is **not just a metaphor—it is a physiological and perceptual reality.** The nervous system does not function in isolation; it is in **constant dialogue with itself, with the environment, and with others.**

1. **Sensory-Motor Resonance** – The nervous system organizes itself **through feedback loops.** Perception and movement are inseparable—our **Shen processes the world based on how we physically interact with it.**
2. **Interpersonal Resonance** – The human nervous system is attuned to **external signals,** from voice tones to facial expressions to environmental cues. **Shen is relational, moving beyond the self into the shared field of experience.**
3. **Embodied Resonance** – Every part of the nervous system is in **communication with every other part.** The Neijing Tu reflects how different Shen interact, revealing that **resonance is not just about connection—it is the foundation of embodied intelligence.**

Mapping the Neijing Tu to The Brain: Resonance

Each **Shen entity** in the Neijing Tu represents **a different aspect of perception, regulation, and resonance**. By mapping these onto the nervous system, we gain insight into how **Shen regulates experience at every level—physical, emotional, and cognitive.**

Shen of the Neijing Tu	Nervous System Function	Resonance & Perception
Yin & Yang (Cerebellum)	Balance, coordination, sensory-motor processing	The foundation of body awareness and movement resonance
Oxherd (Medulla)	Autonomic regulation, breath, survival states	Resonance with internal rhythm, breath, and safety
Weaver (Pons)	Sensory-motor integration, adaptation	Resonance between past experience and present action
Child (Trigeminal Nerve)	Facial expression, emotional response	Resonance through relational attunement, engagement
Buddha (12th Cranial Nerve - Hypoglossal)	Speech, articulation, vocalization	Resonance through voice, self-expression, and communication
Lao Tzu (1st Cranial Nerve - Olfactory)	Intuition, deep sensory perception	Resonance with the unseen, direct knowing beyond words

📌 **Note:** This mapping of the **Shen of the Neijing Tu to the nervous system and evolutionary framework** is part of a **new model** developed through **Neuroaffective Somatics**. As such, there is no external reference beyond my own research, synthesis, and lived experience in this field.

Refining the Shen of Yin & Yang – Cerebellum & Instinctual Balance

PRIMORDIAL

YIN AND YANG

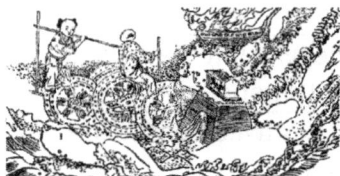

The **cerebellum** governs **balance, proprioception, and the interplay of stillness and motion**—just as **Yin and Yang continuously shift in dynamic equilibrium.** Before conscious thought, before learned movement, the **cerebellum organizes how we exist within gravity.**

This **pre-verbal intelligence** is the foundation for all bodily action. Without it, there is no **fluidity, no stability, no ability to move through space with awareness.**

◆ **Philosophical Insight:** Before cognition, before breath, we are **first moving beings**, shaped by **gravity, weight, and contact with the Earth.**

Aspect	Function in the Body & Nervous System	Embodied Experience
Cerebellum	Coordinates movement, posture, and balance	The body's ability to move fluidly without conscious effort
Yin & Yang	Dynamic interplay of stability (Yin) and motion (Yang)	The unconscious shift between grounding and activation
Instinctual Balance	Pre-verbal awareness of gravity and space	Standing upright without "thinking" about it
Plantar Fascia & Feet	Foundation of bipedal movement	The elasticity that propels the body forward

Evolutionary Alignment: 👣 Homo sapiens –Great Ape

Category	Description
Classification	Genus *Homo*, Species *sapiens*
Embodiment	Feet, Plantar Fascia, Bipedal Movement
Shen Function	Pre-Verbal Knowing, Instinctual Balance
Evolutionary Relevance	The human foot is an evolutionary marvel, balancing stability with adaptation

Why This Matters: The Neijing Tu Depicts a Human, Not Just Any Primate

The **Neijing Tu** does not depict just any living being—it is unmistakably **human**. While all great apes share a common ancestry, humans are unique in **bipedal structure, nervous system complexity, and embodied Shen.**

Unlike other primates, humans:

- **Walk fully upright,** freeing the hands for **expression, creation, and refinement.**
- **Have a highly specialized cerebellum,** fine-tuning **balance, coordination, and movement fluidity.**
- **Experience perception as an alchemical process,** refining **sensory input into wisdom.**

The human body is **not a static vessel** but a **site of transformation, resonance, and Shen cultivation.** The **Neijing Tu** honors this, showing that **internal refinement is inseparable from human embodiment.**

How Yin and Yang in the Neijing Tu Support Nervous System Resonance

1. Yin and Yang Regulate Neural Rhythms

- **Yin (Stillness, Receptivity) → Parasympathetic nervous system** → Supports **rest, repair, and integration.**
- **Yang (Motion, Activation) → Sympathetic nervous system** → Mobilizes **energy and response.**
- **The cerebellum fine-tunes** the balance between **activation and relaxation,** adjusting **muscle tone, posture, and movement.**

When Yin and Yang are responsive to each other, the nervous system can **resonate with external stimuli** without becoming **overwhelmed or rigid.** This allows for **fluid adaptation—** shifting between **rest, action, and integration** without getting stuck in one state.

2. The Cerebellum as a Yin-Yang Integrator

The **Neijing Tu places Yin and Yang at the foundation of transformation,** mirroring the **cerebellum's role in nervous system regulation.**

- **The cerebellum harmonizes activation and relaxation,** preventing movement from becoming **rigid or disconnected.**
- It receives **continuous feedback from the body and environment,** adjusting posture and motion in real-time.

- This supports **resonance with gravity, sensory input, and relational movement**, all essential for **nervous system regulation.**

3. Yin-Yang Balance Prevents Dysregulation

- **When Yin is too strong** → Nervous system **slows down too much** → **Fatigue, dissociation, collapse.**
- **When Yang is too strong** → Nervous system stays in **high activation** → **Anxiety, hypervigilance, rigidity.**
- **When Yin and Yang dynamically adjust to each other** → The nervous system **remains resilient, adaptive, and attuned.**

The Oxherd – Medulla Oblongata & Primal Regulation

THE OXHERD

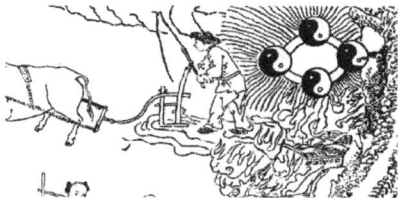

The **medulla oblongata** is the **core of autonomic survival**, governing **breath, heartbeat, and physiological regulation.** It does not operate in isolation—it is **highly responsive to the environment.**

In the **Neijing Tu**, the **Oxherd** represents the **process of refining instinct, not by suppressing it, but by learning how to work with it.** Similarly, nervous system regulation does not happen **by controlling the vagus nerve itself**—it happens **through engagement with space, movement, and** breath.

The **Vagus nerve**, which originates here, **responds to the external world**—just as **TCM** teaches that balance is cultivated through relationship, not isolation.

◆ **Philosophical Insight We cannot Regulate That which is AutoMagic -we can only Resonate**

Oxherd – The Foundation of Primal Regulation

Aspect	Function in the Body & Nervous System	Embodied Experience
Medulla Oblongata	Regulates breath, heartbeat, and autonomic survival states	The unconscious flow of breath and life support
Oxherd	The search for mastery over primal instincts	The tension between impulse and self-regulation
Autonomic Balance	Harmonizes survival responses with conscious awareness	Feeling both grounded and responsive
Diaphragm & Breath	Core interface between voluntary and involuntary control	The ability to shift states through breathwork

Evolutionary Alignment: 🦬 Hominidae (Family) –

Category	Description
Classification	**Family Hominidae** – Great Apes, including humans
Embodiment	Breath, diaphragm, core regulation
Shen Function	Survival Awareness, Social Regulation
Evolutionary Relevance	The medulla ensures survival, while the Vagus nerve adapts us to relationships and space

Why This Matters: The Oxherd, the Medulla, and Nervous System Resonance

The **Oxherd in the Neijing Tu** represents the process of **taming the mind and body**—learning to **engage with instinct without being ruled by it.** This reflects the **medulla's role in regulating survival states without conscious effort.**

1. The Medulla Regulates Core Survival Rhythms
   - Breath, heartbeat, and vagal tone **determine** state regulation.
   - Overactivation leads to chronic stress (sympathetic dominance).
   - Underactivation leads to collapse or disengagement (parasympathetic shutdown).

2. The Medulla as a Bridge Between Instinct & Conscious Control
   - Oxherding is the process of recognizing, not suppressing, instinct.
   - Breath is the only autonomic function we can voluntarily regulate—**this gives access to** state shifts and emotional regulation.

3. Nervous System Balance Requires Environmental Awareness
   - The vagus nerve does not self-regulate—it responds to surroundings.
   - Regulation occurs through engagement with space, rhythm, and breath.
   - This aligns with TCM principles, where health is not just internal but shaped by external Qi and environmental attunement.

How the Oxherd Supports Nervous System Resonance

1. The Medulla Sets the Foundation for Safety & Engagement

   - Autonomic rhythms (breath, heartbeat) create the baseline for nervous system function.
   - Overactivation leads to hypervigilance; underactivation leads to collapse.

2. The Vagus Nerve Listens to the Environment

   - The medulla does not regulate the body alone—it listens to surroundings.
   - Nervous system regulation happens through interaction with external space, breath, and movement.

3. Attunement, Not Control, Creates Resonance

   - The nervous system cannot be "forced" into balance.
   - Resonance occurs when breath, posture, and awareness align with the natural rhythms of the body.

The Weaver – Pons & Sensorimotor Integration

The **pons** is the **bridge between sensation and action**, integrating **movement, balance, and awareness** across the body. It serves as a **relay center** between the brainstem and higher structures, ensuring **fluid coordination of motion, facial expression, and sensory-motor feedback.**

THE WEAVER

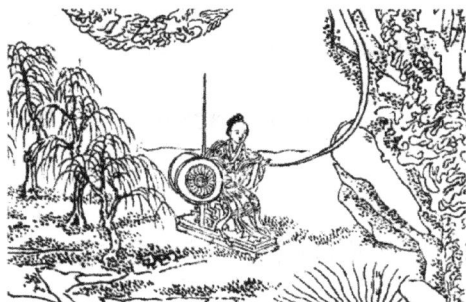

In the **Neijing Tu**, the **Weaver** represents the **intricate dance between perception and response.** Just as the **pons weaves sensory input into coherent movement**, the Weaver harmonizes experience into embodied understanding.

◆ **Philosophical Insight:** There is no movement without sensation, no action without

Weaver – The Foundation of Sensorimotor Integration

Aspect	Function in the Body & Nervous System	Embodied Experience
Pons	Relays sensory and motor signals; coordinates balance and facial expression	The seamless flow between sensation and movement
Weaver	The harmonization of perception and action	The body's ability to adjust fluidly to new experiences
Sensory-Motor Bridge	Regulates balance, coordination, and learned movement	Feeling stable yet adaptable in motion
Facial Expression & Breath	Connects emotion to breath and movement	Expressing without words; responding without hesitation

Evolutionary Alignment: 🕸 Primates (Order) – The Weaving of Experience

Category	Description
Classification	**Order Primates** – The most adaptable mammals
Embodiment	Hands, facial expression, fine motor control
Shen Function	Sensory-Motor Awareness, Adaptation
Evolutionary Relevance	The pons refines movement, allowing complex social and environmental interaction

Why This Matters: The Weaver & Nervous System Resonance

The **pons ensures that movement is never isolated from sensation.** It allows the body to **adjust, refine, and learn**, keeping **action and awareness in sync.**

- The **Weaver in the Neijing Tu** symbolizes this **constant interplay**—the act of shaping raw experience into **fluid, embodied intelligence.**
- **Without this integration, movement is mechanical, perception is fragmented, and expression is disconnected.**

How the Weaver Supports Nervous System Resonance

1. The Pons Bridges Sensory Input & Motor Response

- Sensation informs action—movement refines perception.
- Balance, coordination, and facial expression **all rely on** fluid communication between body and brain.

2. The Pons Allows for Adaptation & Refinement

- It regulates posture, facial engagement, and breath-based expression.
- Attuned responses—not reflexive reactions—create true nervous system resonance.

3. Nervous System Regulation Requires Weaving, Not Just Reacting

- Overstimulation → Sensory overload, uncoordinated movement, or emotional rigidity.
- Understimulation → Loss of adaptability, sluggish response, or disconnection from sensation.
- Integration allows for fluid adjustment—balancing stability with flexibility.

Child – Trigeminal Nerve & Emotional Perception

THE CHILD

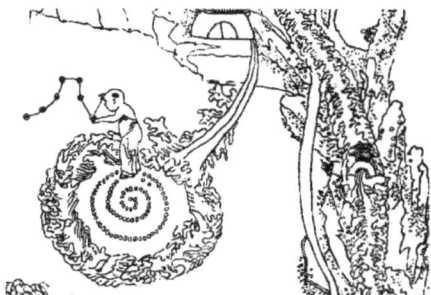

The trigeminal nerve encodes touch, expression, and the felt experience of connection. Like the Child on the Bridge, it links internal awareness to the outer world, bridging sensation, emotion, and the resonance of presence.

The Child on the Star Bridge is, indeed The Inner Child. How lovely is that? Contemplating with this concept will bring forward "Social Engagement" without force.

Child – The Foundation of Emotional Perception

Aspect	Function in the Body & Nervous System	Embodied Experience
Trigeminal Nerve	Governs facial sensation, touch, and jaw movement	The ability to feel and respond before cognition
Child	The raw, unfiltered experience of sensation and emotion	Openness to experience without hesitation
Emotional Reflexes	Early expressions of fear, joy, comfort, and distress	The body's first language—facial expression and breath
Jaw & Mouth	The first interface with nourishment and communication	The ability to receive, express, and shape interaction

Evolutionary Alignment: 👶🏻 Mammalia (Class) – The Birth of Emotional Intelligence

Category	Description
Classification	**Class Mammalia** – Warm-blooded, nurturing, and emotionally responsive species
Embodiment	Face, mouth, breath, early attachment behaviors
Shen Function	Emotional Perception, Early Sensory Awareness
Evolutionary Relevance	The trigeminal nerve allows mammals to sense, nurture, and express through touch and facial feedback

Why This Matters: The Child & Nervous System Resonance

The trigeminal nerve is the first point of contact between sensation and emotional regulation. It allows infants to feel safety, seek connection, and form the foundation of social engagement.

- The Child in the Neijing Tu reflects this early, unfiltered sensory experience.
- Before complex thought, the nervous system regulates through touch, breath, and facial feedback.
- Disruptions in this system can lead to dysregulated emotional response, tension in the jaw, or difficulty processing sensation.

How the Child Supports Nervous System Resonance

1. The Trigeminal Nerve Connects Emotion to Sensation

- Facial expressions are the first form of social and emotional regulation.
- Jaw tension, breath, and facial responsiveness all shape how we feel and express ourselves.

2. Early Sensory Awareness Sets the Foundation for Regulation

- Infants regulate through sensation first, cognition later.
- Breath and facial movement remain lifelong tools for nervous system balance.

3. A Resonating Trigeminal System Supports Social Engagement

- When this system is balanced → Ease of expression, emotional clarity, openness to connection.
- When dysregulated → Jaw tension, shallow breathing, facial rigidity, emotional suppression.
- Breath, sensation, and expression must remain **flexible** for the nervous system to resonate with the external world.

Buddha – Hypoglossal Nerve & The Power of Speech

BUDDHA

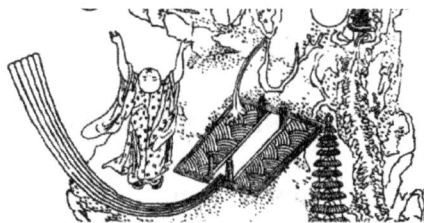

The **hypoglossal nerve (12th cranial nerve)** controls **speech, articulation, and the coordination of the tongue.** It is the bridge between **internal awareness and external expression,** shaping how we bring thought into form.

In the **Neijing Tu**, the **Buddha** represents **the refinement of perception into wisdom.** Just as the **hypoglossal nerve allows us to shape sound into meaning, the Buddha symbolizes the transformation of raw experience into conscious expression.**

◆ **Philosophical Insight:** Speech is not just communication—it is resonance. Words shape reality, defining how we relate to ourselves and the world.

Buddha – The Foundation of Articulation & Expression

Aspect	Function in the Body & Nervous System	Embodied Experience
Hypoglossal Nerve	Controls tongue movement for speech and swallowing	The ability to form words and express meaning
Buddha	The refinement of experience into wisdom	Speech as a bridge between inner knowing and outer reality
Verbal Resonance	The ability to shape and refine expression	Speaking with clarity and intention
Breath & Sound	Regulates vocalization, articulation, and the rhythm of speech	Feeling words as vibrational forces in the body

Evolutionary Alignment: 🧬 Chordata (Phylum) – The Birth of Verbal Communication

Category	Description
Classification	**Phylum Chordata** – Organisms with a nervous system and complex vocalization abilities
Embodiment	Tongue, vocal cords, breath, refined speech
Shen Function	Verbal Intelligence, Expressive Clarity
Evolutionary Relevance	The hypoglossal nerve allows humans to shape complex language, a defining trait of higher cognition

Why This Matters: The Buddha & Nervous System Resonance

The **hypoglossal nerve is not just about speech—it is about resonance.** It determines **how we project, regulate, and refine our voice, shaping both external communication and internal coherence.**

- The **Buddha in the Neijing Tu** represents **the power of refined speech as an act of presence and awareness.**
- **Vocalization is a primary way we regulate the nervous system**, influencing breath, rhythm, and emotional tone.
- **The quality of our speech reflects the state of our nervous system.**

How the Buddha Supports Nervous System Resonance

1. The Hypoglossal Nerve Links Speech to Breath & Nervous System Regulation

- Speech is shaped by the breath—disruptions in breath affect vocal expression.
- The rhythm of speech reflects autonomic balance—fast speech signals activation, slow speech signals relaxation.

2. Verbal Resonance Affects Emotional & Social Regulation

- Tone, pacing, and articulation shape how we are perceived and understood.
- Clear, intentional speech fosters nervous system attunement in relationships.

3. Nervous System Regulation Requires Sound, Not Just Silence

- When verbal expression is blocked → Tension, suppression, emotional stagnation.
- When speech is overactive → Disorganization, nervous chatter, loss of grounding.
- Balanced vocalization allows for calm, intentional resonance within and beyond the body.

Lao Tzu – Olfactory Nerve & Intuitive Perception

LAU TZU

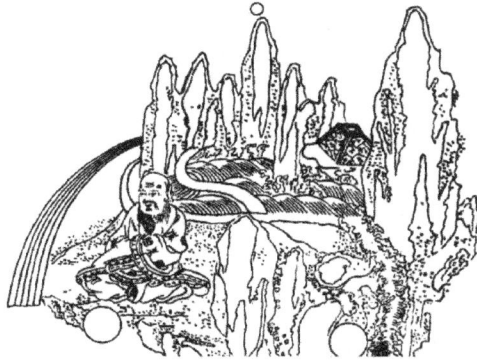

The **olfactory nerve (1st cranial nerve)** governs **smell, direct sensory perception, and deep memory.** Unlike other senses, **olfaction bypasses the thalamus, connecting directly to the limbic system**—the seat of **emotion, instinct, and intuition.**

In the **Neijing Tu, Lao Tzu** represents **the wisdom of direct knowing—the ability to sense without needing to explain.** Just as the **olfactory nerve detects the unseen through scent, Lao Tzu embodies perception that transcends logic.**

◆ **Philosophical Insight:** The deepest truths are not reasoned into existence—they are sensed, lived, and experienced directly.

Lao Tzu – The Foundation of Perception

Aspect	Function in the Body & Nervous System	Embodied Experience
Olfactory Nerve	Detects scent and sends signals directly to the limbic system	The ability to sense before analyzing
Lao Tzu	The embodiment of direct knowing and effortless action	Trusting what is felt beyond words
Intuitive Awareness	Bypasses rational thought to engage deep instinct	Feeling truth as an immediate, wordless experience
Breath & Atmosphere	The quality of air, environment, and presence	The ability to attune to subtle energetic shifts

Evolutionary Alignment: 🌍 Animalia (Kingdom) – The Instinct to Sense & Navigate

Category	Description
Classification	Kingdom Animalia – Organisms that move, adapt, and sense their world
Embodiment	Scent, breath, instinct, environmental awareness
Shen Function	Intuition, Direct Knowing, Unfiltered Perception
Evolutionary Relevance	The olfactory nerve is one of the oldest sensory pathways, ensuring survival through direct environmental attunement

Why This Matters: Lao Tzu & Nervous System Resonance

The **olfactory nerve connects perception directly to emotion and instinct.** It **does not wait for cognitive interpretation—it knows.**

- The **Neijing Tu places Lao Tzu at the level of effortless perception**, where **wisdom arises not from thinking, but from being.**
- **Olfactory input is one of the strongest triggers for memory, emotion, and nervous system response.**
- **The quality of breath, air, and scent directly influences regulation and presence.**

How Lao Tzu Supports Nervous System Resonance

1. The Olfactory Nerve Bypasses Thought to Directly Influence Nervous System State

- Scents can trigger safety, fear, attraction, or calm instantly.
- Breath carries the imprint of presence—how we breathe is how we feel.

2. Direct Perception Shapes Nervous System Adaptability

- Overanalyzing experience disconnects from direct attunement.
- Sensing without needing to explain fosters deep nervous system coherence.

3. Regulation Requires Trusting Sensory Intelligence

- When sensory input is dismissed → Overreliance on logic, loss of instinctive regulation.
- When perception is trusted → Alignment with rhythm, presence, and environmental awareness.
- Nervous system balance is not achieved through control but through deep listening.

Mapping all 12 Cranial Nerves

The following mapping of cranial nerves to the Shen of the organs represents a novel integration of neurophysiology and Daoist energetics. While cranial nerves have been linked to meridians in acupuncture theory, their direct correlation to the Shen of the Zang-Fu is not a traditional model found in classical Chinese medical texts. This framework expands on existing understandings by considering the role of each cranial nerve in perception, movement, and embodied awareness through the Jing-Qi-Shen lens.

RESONATE
EXPERIENCE OF ALL

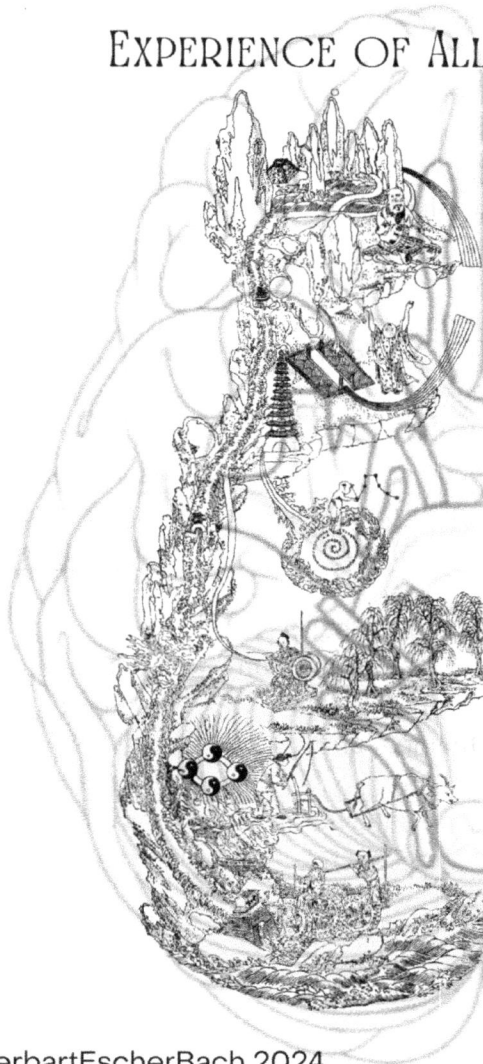

REGULATE
PRIMACY OF VAGUS

olfactory

optic

oculomotor

trochlear

trigeminal

abducens
facial

vestibulochoclear

glossopharyngeal

vagus

hypoglossal

accessory

ZitterbartEscherBach 2024

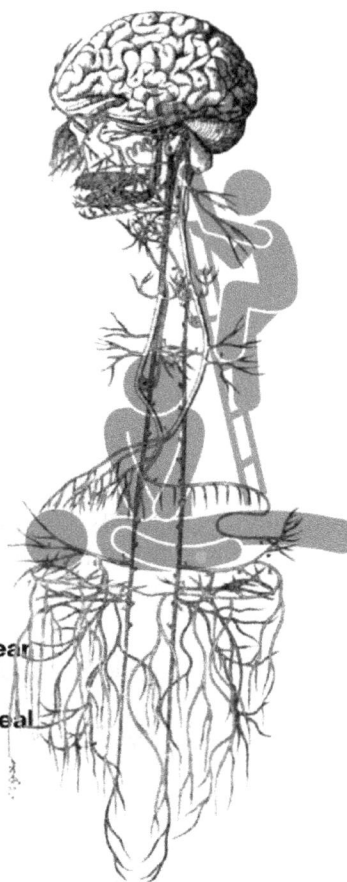

hello@kayteezee.com

Each **cranial nerve (CN I–XII)** plays a role in **perception, movement, and autonomic regulation**. Below, each nerve is described in terms of its **physiological function, its role in perception and movement, and its alignment within the Neuroaffective Somatics.**

Cranial Nerve	Function	Organ (Shen Association)	Shen Expression
Olfactory (I)	Smell, primal sensing	Lung (Po - Corporeal Soul)	Portal to Primordial Perception
Optic (II)	Vision, light processing	Liver (Hun - Ethereal Soul)	Seeing the Origin
Oculomotor (III)	Eye movement, focus	Gallbladder (Courage & Decision-Making)	Axis of Form & Motion
Trochlear (IV)	Eye tracking (superior oblique)	Bladder (Water Memory & Instinct)	Stabilizer of Vision & Balance
Trigeminal (V)	Facial sensation, chewing	Stomach (Yi - Intellect & Processing)	Awareness Through Contact
Abducens (VI)	Eye abduction (lateral rectus)	Small Intestine (Clarity & Discernment)	Tracking the Internal & External
Facial (VII)	Expression, taste (anterior tongue)	Heart (Shen - Spirit & Consciousness)	Emotion as Movement
Vestibulocochlear (VIII)	Hearing, balance	Kidney (Zhi - Will & Deep Knowing)	Tuning to Resonance
Glossopharyngeal (IX)	Swallowing, taste (posterior tongue)	Spleen (Yi - Thought & Integration)	Bridge Between Essence & Voice
Vagus (X)	Parasympathetic regulation, breath, digestion	Pericardium (Shen's Protection & Expression)	Conductor of the Inner Symphony
Accessory (XI)	Neck, shoulders, posture	Triple Burner (Fluid Communication & Regulation)	Structural Integrity of Awareness
Hypoglossal (XII)	Tongue control, speech articulation	Large Intestine (Letting Go & Expression)	Speaking the Internal

Why Map Cranial Nerves to the Shen of the Organs?

Most models of **nervous system regulation** operate within a **binary framework**—a system of **activation vs. inhibition, sympathetic vs. parasympathetic**, or **stress vs. relaxation.** While these approaches capture important aspects of regulation, they **lack a third dimension**—one that accounts for **perception, meaning-making, and the felt experience of awareness itself.**

By introducing **Shen** into the mapping of cranial nerves, this model **moves beyond a binary regulation system** and instead **creates a trine—Jing, Qi, and Shen—where:**

- **Jing (Structure & Physiology)** is the **anatomical function** of each cranial nerve.
- **Qi (Flow & Regulation)** is the **sensorimotor role**—how each nerve mediates movement, awareness, and energetic shifts.
- **Shen (Perceptual Intelligence)** is the **organ's Shen expression**, shaping **not just regulation, but lived experience.**

This **threefold approach** acknowledges that **perception is not passive**—it is an **active, shaping force** in nervous system function. Rather than simply responding to stimuli through excitation or inhibition, the **body-mind system organizes itself through resonance, coherence, and meaning.**

In this way, **Shen completes the triad**, transforming the cranial nerves from **mechanical regulators into pathways of embodied awareness.**

1. **Olfactory Nerve (CN I) – Smell – Portal to Primordial Perception**
   - **Physiological function:** Governs smell, linking directly to memory, emotion, and breath regulation.
   - **Energetic and sensorimotor mapping:** Smell is the first threshold of perception, guiding awareness toward visceral states, safety, and intuition. It is deeply tied to the breath cycle and primal responses.
   - **Shen correspondence: Lung (Po – Corporeal Soul)** – The Po governs breath and instinctual knowing, linking olfactory perception to survival, memory, and the embodied present moment.
2. **Optic Nerve (CN II) – Vision – Seeing the Origin**
   - **Physiological function:** Transmits visual information, allowing spatial awareness, motor control, and predictive movement.
   - **Energetic and sensorimotor mapping:** Vision acts as a bridge between external perception and internal knowing, influencing clarity, foresight, and orientation.
   - **Shen correspondence: Liver (Hun – Ethereal Soul)** – The Liver "opens to the eyes," and the Hun governs vision, dreaming, and the capacity to see beyond the present moment.
3. **Oculomotor Nerve (CN III) – Eye Movement – Axis of Form & Motion**
   - **Physiological function:** Controls eye positioning and pupil dilation, allowing focus and gaze stability.
   - **Energetic and sensorimotor mapping:** Regulates intent and directionality, stabilizing movement and energy flow.

- Shen correspondence: Gallbladder (Decision-Making & Courage) – The Gallbladder meridian influences decisiveness and movement initiation, mirroring the role of the oculomotor nerve in maintaining direction and control.

4. **Trochlear Nerve (CN IV) – Eye Tracking – Stabilizer of Vision & Balance**
   - **Physiological function:** Governs superior oblique muscle function, critical for depth perception and head positioning.
   - **Energetic and sensorimotor mapping:** Ensures equilibrium between inner and outer perception, maintaining **visual stability and spatial balance**.
   - **Shen correspondence: Bladder (Water Memory & Instinct)** – The Bladder meridian governs spinal alignment, postural stability, and the ability to track movement fluidly across space.

5. **Trigeminal Nerve (CN V) – Facial Sensation & Chewing – Awareness Through Contact**
   - **Physiological function:** The largest cranial nerve, responsible for facial sensation and mastication.
   - **Energetic and sensorimotor mapping:** Mediates physical and energetic contact with the world, integrating touch, proprioception, and nourishment.
   - **Shen correspondence: Stomach (Yi – Thought & Processing)** – The Stomach is responsible for nourishment and the Yi governs intellect, digestion (both physical and mental), and our interaction with the material world.

6. **Abducens Nerve (CN VI) – Lateral Eye Movement – Tracking the Internal & External**
   - **Physiological function:** Enables lateral gaze, coordinating head and eye movement for orientation.
   - **Energetic and sensorimotor mapping:** Aligns vision with shifting environmental inputs, regulating adaptability.
   - **Shen correspondence: Small Intestine (Clarity & Discernment)** – The Small Intestine sorts pure from impure, reflecting this nerve's role in discriminating visual input and tracking shifts in awareness.

7. **Facial Nerve (CN VII) – Expression & Taste – Emotion as Movement**
   - **Physiological function:** Controls facial expressions and anterior tongue taste.
   - **Energetic and sensorimotor mapping:** Governs **emotional embodiment**, translating inner states into visible expressions and social cues.
   - **Shen correspondence: Heart (Shen – Spirit & Consciousness)** – The Heart governs Shen, and the face reflects the **inner radiance of the spirit.**

8. **Vestibulocochlear Nerve (CN VIII) – Hearing & Balance – Tuning to Resonance**
   - **Physiological function:** Regulates auditory perception and equilibrium, coordinating movement with sound.
   - **Energetic and sensorimotor mapping:** Governs harmony between **inner stillness and outer movement**, attuning the nervous system to resonance.
   - **Shen correspondence: Kidney (Zhi – Will & Deep Knowing)** – The Kidneys govern the ears, reflecting the **deep listening and wisdom of the Zhi.**

9. **Glossopharyngeal Nerve (CN IX) – Swallowing & Taste – Bridge Between Essence & Voice**
   - **Physiological function:** Mediates swallowing, posterior tongue taste, and blood pressure regulation.
   - **Energetic and sensorimotor mapping:** Aligns **ingestion with refinement**, forming a threshold where material meets energetic transformation.

- o **Shen correspondence: Spleen (Yi – Thought & Integration)** – The Spleen processes nourishment (physical and mental), refining substance into energy.
- o

10. **Vagus Nerve (CN X) – Autonomic Regulation & Voice – Conductor of the Inner Symphony**
    - o **Physiological function:** Regulates parasympathetic tone, digestion, respiration, and vocalization.
    - o **Energetic and sensorimotor mapping:** Governs **Qi flow through the body's deepest channels**, uniting breath, voice, and visceral function.
    - o **Shen correspondence: Pericardium (Shen's Protection & Expression)** – The Pericardium governs **emotional regulation and heart-lung balance**, mirroring the Vagus Nerve's role in safety and connection.

11. **Accessory Nerve (CN XI) – Neck & Shoulder Movement – Structural Integrity of Awareness**

    - o **Physiological function:** Controls head rotation and shoulder elevation.
    - o **Energetic and sensorimotor mapping:** The structural **pillar of upper-body alignment**, ensuring posture reflects inner integrity.
    - o **Shen correspondence: Triple Burner (Fluid Communication & Regulation)** – The Triple Burner coordinates **energetic and physical structure** across the body.

12. **Hypoglossal Nerve (CN XII) – Tongue Control – Verbal expression**

    - o **Physiological function:** Regulates tongue positioning for speech and swallowing.
    - o **Energetic and sensorimotor mapping:** Governs **verbal expression and articulation**, translating thought into **spoken resonance.**
    - o **Shen correspondence: Large Intestine (Letting Go & Expression)** – The Large Intestine governs **release and clarity**, mirroring the tongue's role in **verbalization and refinement of ideas.**

How to Engage with This Model

In the body, these three aspects—**Physiological Function, Energetic and Sensorimotor Mapping, and Shen Correspondence**—are **stacked from the bottom up**, mirroring the **Jing-Qi-Shen structure of the Neijing Tu.**

- **Physiological Function (Jing)** corresponds to **the base of the Neijing Tu**, representing the **structural and biological foundation** of each cranial nerve. This is the tangible, physical aspect—what the nerve controls in terms of **sensation, movement, and autonomic regulation.**
- **Energetic and Sensorimotor Mapping (Qi)** reflects **the middle section of the Neijing Tu**, where physiological processes begin to influence **perception, adaptation, and movement.** This is the **functional intelligence** of the system—the way the nerve shapes **how we orient ourselves, respond, and integrate sensory experience.**

- **Shen Correspondence (Shen)** sits **at the top**, aligning with the **subtle, perceptual, and archetypal influences** of the nervous system. This level connects **each cranial nerve to the Shen of the organ it corresponds with**, highlighting the **cognitive, emotional, and spiritual resonance** embedded within its function.

This structure shifts the cranial nerves from being seen as **isolated anatomical parts** to **dynamic perceptual gateways** that shape how we experience and navigate the world.

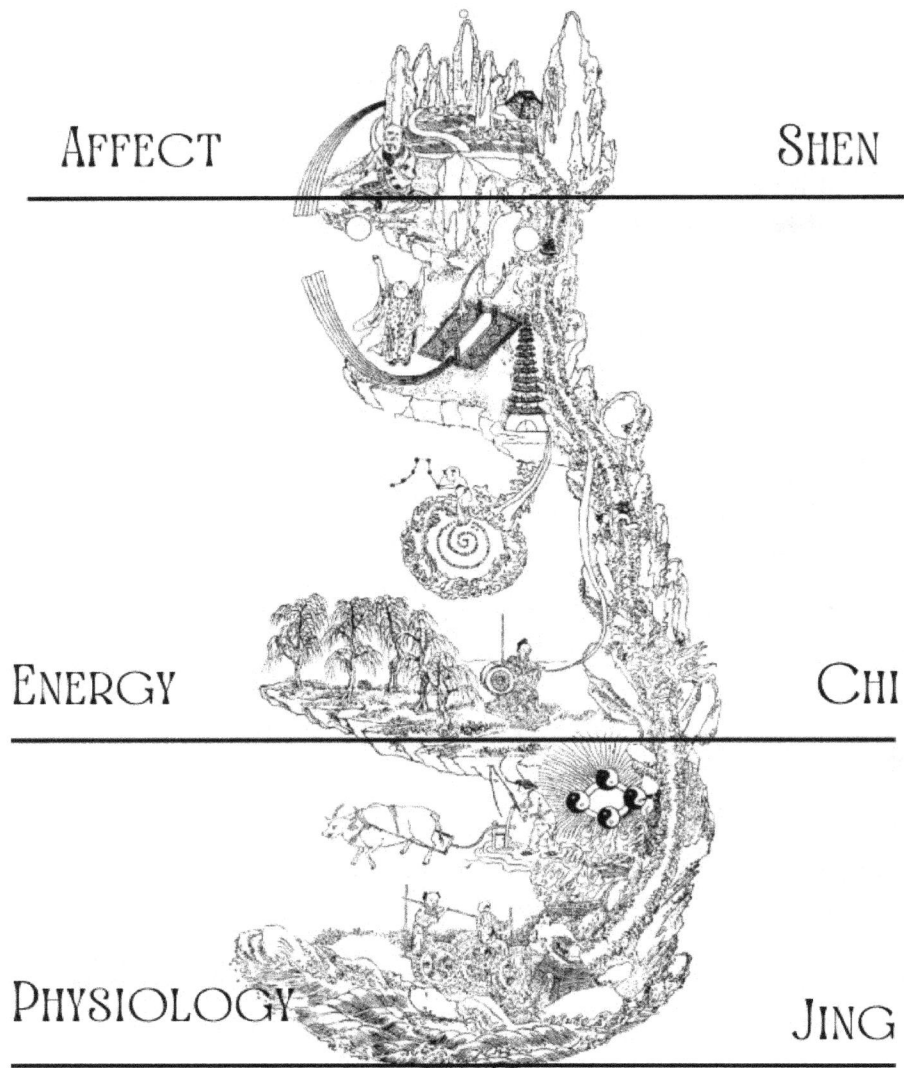

AFFECT   SHEN

ENERGY   CHI

PHYSIOLOGY   JING

Your Body Ba Gua: The Three Dantian, The Eight Extraordinary Vessels, and The Immortals

The Eight Extraordinary Vessels: The Original Currents of Inheritance

Before we develop meridians, before we form identity, and before we take our first breath, we have the **Eight Extraordinary Vessels**—the deepest energetic structures of the body. These vessels are **not like the primary meridians**, which govern daily Qi flow. Instead, they are **pre-birth currents of formation**, shaping:

- **Jing** (Essence): How we inherit ancestral patterns (lineage, genetic imprint, deep structure).
- **Qi** (Vital Energy): How we hold and adapt memory in the body (belonging, fascia, somatic experience).
- **Shen** (Spirit): How we transmit wisdom across time (teaching lines, perception, embodied intelligence).

The Extraordinary Vessels predate individuality, forming the underlying matrix that supports movement, perception, and transformation.

Why Are They Called "Extraordinary"?

Unlike the 12 meridians, which regulate organ function and daily cycles, the Extraordinary Vessels function as reservoirs of deeper intelligence:

1. Store Ancestral & Prenatal Qi – The energy we receive before birth, shaping our structural tendencies.
2. Govern Long-Term Cycles of Growth – They regulate lifelong shifts, beyond momentary fluctuations.
3. Support Adaptation & Evolution – Holding inherited patterns while also enabling transformation.
4. Exist in a State of Superposition – These vessels precede individual form, aligning with wave functions rather than fixed structures. Ancient Daoists understood these as quantum-like currents of potentiality.

If the **12 meridians are like rivers**, distributing **Qi**, then the **Extraordinary Vessels are the oceans and deep currents**, holding the original flow of life itself.

EPIGENETICS

ZitterbartEscherBach

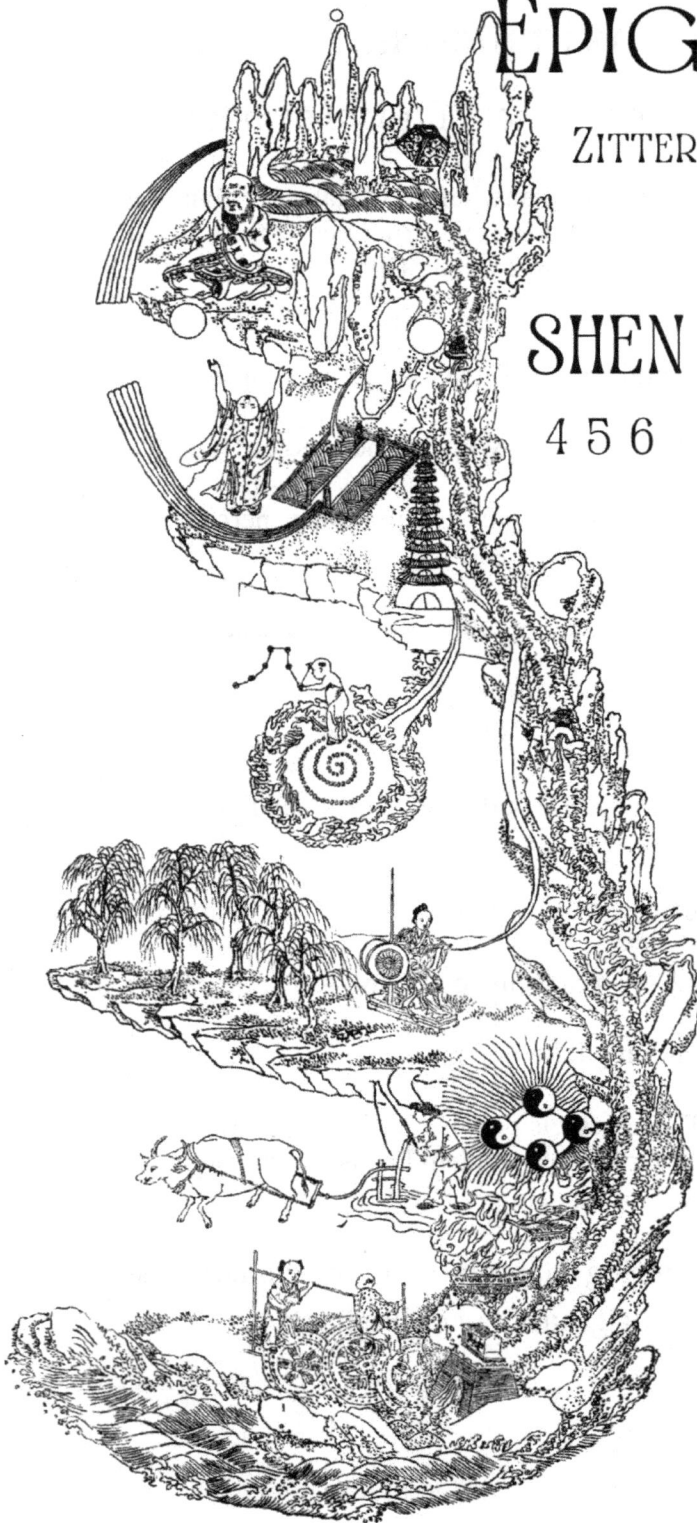

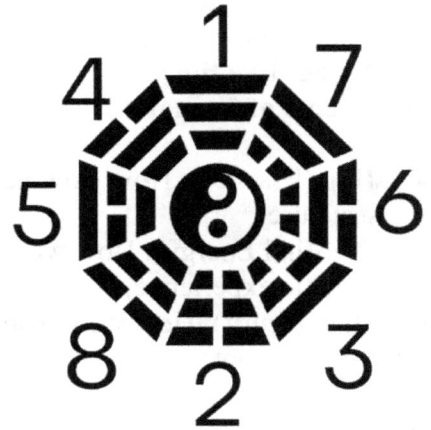

SHEN

4 5 6

CHI

7 8

JING

1 2 3

Definition & Description of the Fu Xi (Earlier Heaven) Bagua

Believe it or not, there is more than one Bagua!. The version I'm using here is the The **Fu Xi (伏羲) or Earlier Heaven (Xiān Tiān 先天) Bagua.** This is an **archetypal arrangement** of the eight trigrams (Ba Gua) that represents **primordial order, cosmic balance, and the unchanging structure of the Dao** before manifestation.

This sequence is often considered the **pure, undisturbed state of reality**—a resonance-based map rather than one focused on human experience or transformation.

Core Aspects of Fu Xi Bagua:

1. **Primordial Equilibrium:**
   o This sequence is not about movement but **resonance**—it reflects the **Dao in its perfect harmony**.
   o Unlike the Later Heaven sequence (which relates to cycles and change), Fu Xi's arrangement **describes fundamental forces in balance before time, space, and cycles emerge.**
2. **Yin-Yang Pairing:**
   o **Each trigram is placed** in opposition to its natural pair**, creating a** harmonic structure of complementary forces.
   o **Example:** Heaven (☰) is opposite Earth (☷), Water (☵) is opposite Fire (☲), etc.
3. **Cosmic Perspective:**
   o This ordering is less about practical applications like Feng Shui or internal alchemy and more about understanding how reality emerges from undivided unity.
   o Shen (Spirit) is the organizing principle—it emphasizes perception, awareness, and attunement to the Dao rather than external action.
4. **Symbolism of the Arrangement:**
   o Heaven (☰) at the top & Earth (☷) at the bottom → **The ultimate** Yang-Yin polarity **structuring all existence.**
   o Thunder (☳) and Wind (☴) on the sides → **Represent the** first movements within stillness, **the emergence of form.**
   o Fire (☲) and Water (☵) across from each other → **The** active alchemical interplay of Yin and Yang in motion.
   o Lake (☱) and Mountain (☶) at the last positions → **Represent** stabilization and return to harmony.

The Three Ancestries: An Extraordinary Framework for Understanding Inheritance & Evolution

The **Three Ancestries** describe the **continuum of inheritance, adaptation, and self-integration**, weaving through **Jing (Essence), Qi (Vital Energy), and Shen (Spirit).** These form the foundation of **how we receive, interact with, and evolve our embodied experience**: The Ancestries are in order, but the Vessels Weave – how cool is that?

I, personally, experience much of this contemplation as happening in/through the Weaver and how she connects us to our ancestors and the cosmos.

1st Ancestry: Jing – The Deep Blueprint (1,2,3)

- **The inherited map** → What we are given.
- Governed by **Chong Mai, Ren Mai, and Du Mai**, this is the realm of **deep genetic imprinting, prenatal energy, and structural integrity.**
- Jing determines **lifespan, physical constitution, and ancestral tendencies.**

2nd Ancestry: Qi – The Adaptation to Life (7,8)

- **The way we engage with life** → What we adapt to.
- Governed by **Yang Wei Mai & Yin Wei Mai**, this is the realm of **relational dynamics, resilience, and sensory-motor intelligence.**
- Qi governs **how we respond to life's cycles, heal, and transform through experience.**

3rd Ancestry: Shen – The Integration & Weaver (4,5,6)

- **The story we create** → How we integrate and evolve.
- Governed by **Yin Qiao, Yang Qiao, and Dai Mai**, this is the realm of **conscious embodiment, perceptual intelligence, and meaning making.**
- Shen determines **how we shape our personal myth, store trauma, and release inherited patterns.**

These Three Ancestries **are not linear** but function as a **fractal, spiraling continuum**, constantly reshaping itself.

Like **fascia**, these vessels do not simply **transport energy**—they create a **living web where movement, memory, and response** are continuously reshaped.

Epigenetics & Tensegrity: The Living Field of Inheritance

The Extraordinary Vessels mediate how inherited structure (Jing), lived adaptation (Qi), and perceptual intelligence (Shen) shape our embodied experience. (Rossi, 2007)

Jing & Shen as Fixed Anchors

- **Jing (Deep Blueprint)** → Genetic inheritance, pre-birth imprints, biological potential.
- **Shen (Perceptual Field)** → The overarching intelligence that interprets experience and organizes meaning.
- These **do not change easily**—they create the foundation for our **physical form (Jing) and perceptual tendencies (Shen).**

Qi as the Adaptive Force

- **Qi is the flexible medium that integrates experience.**
- It responds to **life events, relational patterns, trauma, healing, and regulation.**
- This is where **change happens**—Qi can **modify how Jing expresses itself and how Shen integrates perception.**

Tensegrity in the Extraordinary Vessels

- The **fixed nature** of **Jing & Shen** provides **stability.**
- The **fluid nature** of **Qi** allows for **adaptive self-regulation.**
- **Tensegrity arises when these forces interact dynamically, rather than becoming locked or collapsed.**

Tensegrity provides grounding in Lived Experience

The Three Dantian: Aligning Trigrams, Vessels, and the Immortals

As you recall, the **Three Dantian** represent the body's **three centers of transformation**, aligned with:

1. Lower Dantian (Jing / Earth / Body) – The deep reservoir of ancestral Qi, survival intelligence, and genetic inheritance.
2. Middle Dantian (Qi / Human / Breath) – The realm of relational energy, adaptation, and sensory-motor response.
3. Upper Dantian (Shen / Heaven / Mind-Spirit) – The space of perception, imagination, and consciousness.

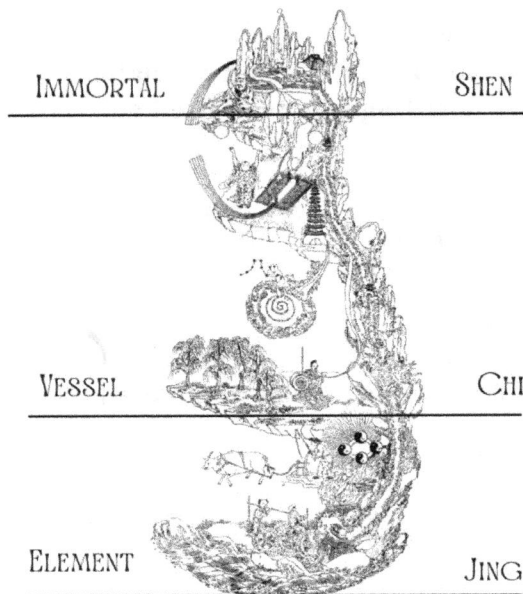

In this system:

- **Jing** aligns to the **Element** (Trigram).
- **Qi** aligns to the **Extraordinary Vessel**.
- **Shen** aligns to the **Immortal (Perceptual Intelligence)**.

This **vertical mapping** transforms the **Ba Gua into an embodied system**, grounding the **abstract symbols** of the **I Ching into the body's structure, movement, and perception.**

We are going to use the Immortals to Bridge

The Eight Immortals are Shen in this System

The **Eight Immortals (八仙, Bāxiān)** are legendary figures in **Taoist folklore**, each representing different aspects of **spiritual transcendence, human virtues, and esoteric wisdom**. They are often depicted together, symbolizing the **harmony of different paths to enlightenment**. They were **widely venerated in Chinese culture**, inspiring **literature, art, theater, and Daoist spiritual practices**.

Historically, the Immortals are the source of Culture. Evolutionarily, then, they represent the connection we have to the Animal Kingdom. We are, after all, Bipedal Great Apes.

Attributes

Each Immortal carries a **unique object (法器, fǎqì)** that signifies their **powers, virtues, or method of immortality**. Their stories reflect **Taoist principles of balance, transformation, and the pursuit of harmony with the Dao (道)**.

Lu Dongbin - Scholar-sage of wisdom and inner alchemy. **Sword**
He Xiangu - Maiden of health and natural vitality. **Lotus Flower**
Zhang Guolao - Alchemist of innovation and resilience. **Drum & Mallets**
Lan Caihe - Mystic of spontaneity and simplicity. **Flowers**
Zhongli Quan - Healer and master of transformation. **Fan**
Cao Guojiu - Guide of discipline and helpful connections. **Jade Tablet**
Han Xiangzi - Artist of creativity and harmony. **Flute**
Li Tieguai - Compassionate wanderer aiding the sick and needy. **Iron Crutch**

How to Contemplate This Model

This system maps each **trigram** to an **Element, an Extraordinary Vessel, and an Immortal**, allowing for multiple entry points into the material. Whether someone resonates more with **mythology (Immortals), physiology (Vessels), or energetic principles (Elements)**, this framework offers a way to engage with the concepts in a way that best aligns with their preferences.

What Makes This Approach Unique?

1. **It Creates a Vertical, Embodied Model**
   o Most traditional **I Ching** or **Ba Gua** interpretations focus on the trigrams as abstract symbols or fortune-telling tools.
   o This system **grounds them in the body**, making the **bottom line** the **core principle**, the **middle line** the **physiological structure**, and the **top line** the **perceptual/spiritual influence**.
   o This mirrors the **Three Dantian model** (Jing → Qi → Shen) but applies it directly to **Neuroaffective Somatics.**

2. **It Integrates the Extraordinary Vessels**
   o The **Extraordinary Vessels (Qi Jing Ba Mai)** are **rarely mapped** to the Ba Gua in this way.
   o Most TCM (Traditional Chinese Medicine) approaches treat them as **deep reservoirs of Qi**, while this model treats them as **structural currents of perception, inheritance, and movement.**
   o This links **the nervous system, fascia, and Daoist alchemy** in a way that's **both somatic and symbolic.**

3. **It Brings in Shen (Immortal/Perceptual Intelligence)**
   o The **Eight Immortals** are rarely used as **a living cognitive framework**—here, they act as **Shen** (perceptual archetypes), influencing how we experience reality.
   o This shifts **the Trigrams** from static symbols into **embodied, living processes** that evolve through **perception, physiology, and meaning.**

4. **It Bridges Classical Chinese Thought with Neuroscience & Somatics**
   o Instead of separating **Ba Gua, TCM, and trauma-informed somatics**, this model **unifies** them into a **practical contemplation tool.**
   o It shows **how perception (Shen), embodiment (Jing), and transformation (Qi) are constantly shaping our experience of self and space.**

Why This Matters

Instead of asking, "What does this Trigram predict?", this system asks:

- How does this Trigram structure my perception and embodiment?
- Where do I experience its influence in my nervous system, posture, and movement?
- How does my relationship with this system reflect my lived experience?

This makes it **not just a theoretical framework, but a practice of embodied self-inquiry**—something rarely seen in either **traditional Daoism** or **modern somatic work**.

A note from Katie: Along with the literature and historic resources I have access to, I used a Chinese LLM to ensure cultural and conceptual alignment.

Mapping the Extraordinary Vessels, Trigrams, and Immortals

Trigram	Extraordinary Vessel (Qi / Structure)	Immortal (Shen / Perception)	Element (Jing / Body)
Qian ☰ (Heaven)	Du Mai (Governing Vessel)	Lü Dongbin (Scholar-Sage)	Metal
Kun ☷ (Earth)	Ren Mai (Conception Vessel)	He Xiangu (Immortal Maiden)	Earth
Zhen ☳ (Thunder)	Yang Wei Mai (Yang Linking Vessel)	Zhang Guolao (Mystic Alchemist)	Wood
Xun ☴ (Wind)	Dai Mai (Belt Vessel)	Cao Guojiu (Noble Patron)	Wood
Li ☲ (Fire)	Chong Mai (Penetrating Vessel)	Zhongli Quan (General-Healer)	Fire
Kan ☵ (Water)	Yin Wei Mai (Yin Linking Vessel)	Lan Caihe (Androgynous Wanderer)	Water
Dui ☱ (Lake)	Yang Qiao Mai (Yang Heel Vessel)	Han Xiangzi (Daoist Musician)	Metal
Gen ☶ (Mountain)	Yin Qiao Mai (Yin Heel Vessel)	Li Tieguai (Iron-Crutch Wanderer)	Earth

Qian ☰ (Heaven) – The Nervous System & The Scholar's Path

In the framework of **Neuroaffective Somatics**, each trigram from the **Bagua (八卦)** is mapped to **Extraordinary Vessels**, which govern deep nervous system regulation and transformation. The trigram **Qian ☰ (Heaven)** corresponds to the **Du Mai (Governing Vessel)**, the body's central channel of structural integrity and leadership.

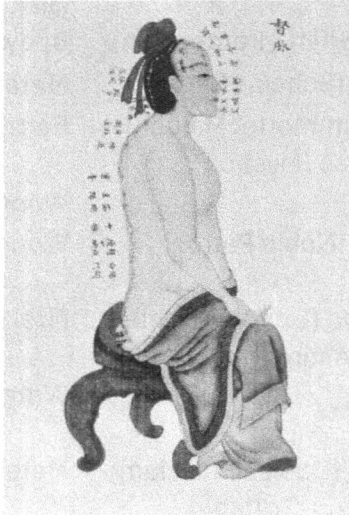

This pairing is associated with **strength, clarity, and resilience**, reflected both in physical postural alignment and in cognitive mastery. The legendary Taoist **Immortal Lü Dongbin** serves as the **Shen (Spirit Influence)** for this system, representing **wisdom, discernment, and the path of self-mastery**.

Understanding this system provides **insight into how perception (Afferent) and action (Efferent) interact**, shaping both our nervous system function and our approach to learning, leadership, and endurance. The tables below summarize its key attributes:

Note: The Art in this section is all from Wiki Commons.

Qian ☰ (Heaven)	Details
Element	Metal
Direction	Northwest
Attributes	Strength, initiation, leadership, clarity, endurance
Feng Shui Associations	Sky, expansive views, high places, open spaces, minimalism, metals
Feng Shui Considerations	- Create Open Space – High ceilings, uncluttered areas, clean lines enhance clarity.
	- Use Metal Elements – Bells, swords, minimalist metal decor reinforce strength.
	- Align Work & Study Areas – Place desks in positions of command and perspective.
	- Symbolic Sword – A reminder of discernment and wisdom, whether literal or figurative.

Du Mai (Governing Vessel) – The Pillar of Inheritance

Du Mai (Governing Vessel)	Nervous System
Function	Governs Yang energy, vitality, and upward movement. Regulates the nervous system, postural integrity, and spinal alignment.
Lineage	The first organizing structure of the nervous system, shaping posture, movement, and resilience.
Belonging	Acts as the spine of embodied presence, regulating autonomy, strength, and self-direction. A well-regulated Du Mai ensures stability, while a disrupted one may lead to postural collapse or loss of direction.
Teaching Line	The path of self-mastery—cultivated by sages and martial artists. Teaches sovereignty, leadership, and endurance through discipline and inner alignment.

Lü Dongbin (呂洞賓) – The Scholar-Sage

Lü Dongbin	Shen
Role	Patron of scholars, poets, and martial artists; associated with inner alchemy and wisdom.
Cultural Significance	- One of the most venerated Immortals. - Left behind worldly ambitions to study Daoist alchemy. - Known for encounters with demons and spirits, testing his virtue and wisdom.
Symbol	Sword of Wisdom – Represents his power to dispel ignorance and illusion.
Key Legend	- Tested 10 times by Zhongli Quan before achieving immortality. - Became a wandering sage, teaching inner alchemy and transformation.

Balance & Imbalance of the Qian/Du Mai System

The **Qian/Du Mai pairing** embodies the **structural and energetic axis of leadership, clarity, and self-mastery**. When in balance, it cultivates **mental precision, resilience, and embodied wisdom**—the ability to stand firm while remaining adaptable.

However, **too much structure** can lead to **rigidity and over-intellectualization**, while **too little** can result in **collapse, loss of direction, or dissociation**. The nervous system, like the spine itself, thrives on **dynamic equilibrium**—strong yet fluid, disciplined yet open.

By attuning to **Qian's expansive clarity** and **Du Mai's spine of presence**, we learn to **hold integrity without rigidity** and **lead without forcing control**. Mastery is not about domination—it is about alignment with the natural unfolding of experience.

Qian ☰ / Du Mai State	Effects
Excess (Overactive State)	- Rigid Thinking & Over-Control – Inability to adapt. - Hypervigilance – Overactive nervous system, always "on guard." - Over-Intellectualization – Prioritizing logic over emotion.
Deficiency (Weakened State)	- Collapse & Weak Boundaries – Loss of physical and mental uprightness. - Disorientation – Difficulty sensing direction or purpose. - Dissociation & Energy Drain – Feeling disconnected from one's own power.
Balanced State (Ideal Expression)	- Embodied Wisdom – A sharp mind with fluid movement. - Clarity in Action – The ability to stand firm while remaining adaptable. - Integrity & Leadership – The spine as a symbol of truth and resilience.

Applying the Qian/Du Mai Pairing in Practice

Influence	Details
Afferent (Perception) – Lü Dongbin's Shen Influence	- Wisdom & Discernment – Cutting through misinformation, refining awareness. - Mental Agility – Learning, pattern recognition, adaptability. - Resilience – Facing intellectual, emotional, and physical challenges.
Efferent (Action) – Du Mai's Stru	- Postural Sovereignty – How you hold yourself reflects internal alignment. - Autonomic Nervous System Regulation – Balancing activation and relaxation. - Longevity Practices – Strengthening the spine, breathwork, uprightness.

Kun ☷ (Earth) – The Conception Vessel & The Immortal Maiden

In the framework of **Neuroaffective Somatics**, each trigram from the **Bagua (八卦)** is mapped to an **Extraordinary Vessel**, which governs deep **physiological and energetic regulation**. The trigram **Kun ☷ (Earth)** corresponds to the **Ren Mai (Conception Vessel)**, the body's **central channel for nourishment, reproductive vitality, and emotional security**.

This pairing is associated with **softness, patience, and deep support**, expressed through both **physical fertility and emotional containment**. The legendary Taoist **Immortal He Xiangu** serves as the **Shen (Spirit Influence)** for this system, representing **self-compassion, healing through receptivity, and alignment with natural rhythms**.

Understanding this system provides insight into **how we receive and integrate care**, shaping both our **hormonal health and emotional resilience**. The tables below summarize its key attributes:

Note: The art in this section is from **WikiCommons**

Kun ☷ (Earth) – The Ground of Support

Kun ☷ (Earth)	Details
Element	Earth
Direction	Southwest
Attributes	Receptivity, nourishment, patience, deep support, embodiment
Feng Shui Associations	Mother energy, fertile soil, grounding, home, safety, adaptability
	- Create a Nurturing Space – Soft, rounded furniture, warm colors, and natural materials (clay, ceramics) enhance receptivity.
	- Supportive Grounding – Thick rugs, floor seating, or comfortable resting areas reinforce stability and trust.
	- Symbolic Lotus – A reminder of resilience and growth through nourishment, whether literal (plants, flowers) or metaphorical (art, imagery).
Feng Shui Considerations	- Soften Lighting & Textures – Gentle illumination and tactile fabrics encourage relaxation and Yin energy.

Ren Mai (Conception Vessel) – The River of Self-Compassion

Ren Mai (Conception Vessel)	Reproductive & Emotional System
Function	Governs Yin energy, reproductive health, fertility, and emotional nourishment.
	- The Ren Mai is the holding field of gestation, the matrix of Yin that nurtures and sustains life.
	- It governs how we receive nourishment, how we feel connected, and how we learn to trust.
Lineage – The First Embrace	- Before birth, it is the amniotic field that contains us, the ocean of being before we are separate.
	- In fascia, the Ren Mai relates to the fluid balance of the body, regulating moisture, adaptability, and hormonal intelligence.
	- It holds the experience of safety, comfort, and being welcomed into existence.
Belonging – The River of Self-Compassion	- A strong Ren Mai allows for emotional warmth and connection, while a disrupted one may lead to difficulty receiving love, hormonal imbalances, or struggles with fertility.
	- The Ren Mai transmits the teachings of mothering, self-compassion, and deep receptivity.
	- It is the line of healers, caregivers, and those who cultivate Yin wisdom.
Teaching Line – The Line of Nourishment & Care	- Its lessons are learned through softness, allowing, and the acceptance of being held.

He Xiangu (何仙姑) – The Immortal Maiden

He Xiangu	Shen
Role	Patron of health, vitality, and feminine wisdom; represents natural beauty and purity.
	- The only female among the Eight Immortals, she embodies gentleness, healing, and connection to nature.
	- In some legends, she was a real historical figure during the Tang Dynasty.
	- She was known for her vegetarian diet, emphasizing balance between the body, spirit, and nature.
Cultural Significance	Lotus Flower – Represents purity, compassion, and spiritual elevation.
Symbol	- At age 14, she had a vision where an immortal taught her to eat powdered mica, which made her light as a feather and free from hunger.
	- She eventually ascended to the heavens, leaving only a lotus flower behind.
Key Legend	

Balance & Imbalance of the Kun/Ren Mai System

The **Kun/Ren Mai pairing** embodies **nourishment, receptivity, and deep emotional grounding**. When in balance, it fosters **a strong sense of belonging, self-compassion, and the ability to receive life with ease**.

However, **excess receptivity** can lead to **over-accommodation, emotional overwhelm, or lack of boundaries**, while **too little receptivity** results in **difficulty trusting, disconnection from the body, and resistance to rest**. The body's **fluid balance, fertility, and Yin containment** must be **stable yet adaptive**—just like the Earth itself.

By attuning to **Kun's deep support** and **Ren Mai's flowing nourishment**, we learn to **honor our natural cycles, embrace Yin wisdom, and cultivate a deep sense of trust in both our bodies and emotions**.

Balance & Imbalance

Kun ☷ / Ren Mai State	Effects
Excess (Overactive State)	- Over-Accommodation & Lack of Boundaries – Always caring for others, neglecting the self. - Emotional Overwhelm – Feeling overly sensitive, easily drained, or overly attached to external validation. - Fluid Retention & Hormonal Imbalance – The body "holding on" instead of processing freely.
Deficiency (Weakened State)	- Lack of Safety & Emotional Disconnection – Difficulty feeling at home in the body or trusting relationships. - Dissociation from Needs – Ignoring hunger, exhaustion, or reproductive health. - Resistance to Rest – Feeling guilty or uneasy when not being productive.
Balanced State (Ideal Expression)	- Rooted & Receptive – Able to receive love, care, and nourishment without fear or guilt. - Deeply Present in the Body – Feeling at home within oneself, honoring natural cycles and bodily needs. - Emotional & Hormonal Resilience – Grounded, stable, and able to navigate relationships without losing center.

Applying the Kun/Ren Mai Pairing in Practice

Influence	Details
Afferent (Perception) – He Xiangu's Shen Influence	- Feminine Wisdom & Nourishment – How we receive, absorb, and integrate sustenance (physical, emotional, intellectual). - Healing through Receptivity – The ability to soften into care, rather than force solutions. - Resonance with Natural Rhythms – Aligning with menstrual cycles, hormonal balance, and the wisdom of the body. - Trust in One's Own Body & Needs – Understanding hunger, fertility, fatigue, and restoration.
Efferent (Action) – Ren Mai's Structural Expression	- Self-Compassion as a Practice – Cultivating inner kindness and emotional regulation. - Stability through Adaptability – Learning to be supported without rigidity.

Zhen ☳ (Thunder) – The Yang Linking Vessel & The Mystic Alchemist

In the framework of **Neuroaffective Somatics**, each trigram from the **Bagua (八卦)** is mapped to an **Extraordinary Vessel**, which governs deep **physiological and energetic regulation**. The trigram **Zhen ☳ (Thunder)** corresponds to the **Yang Wei Mai (Yang Linking Vessel)**, the body's **first response system**, organizing **Yang energy for movement, adaptability, and immune resilience**.

This pairing is associated with **boldness, initiation, and the body's ability to react to external stimuli**, whether through **immune function, stress response, or dynamic movement**. The legendary Taoist **Immortal Zhang Guolao** serves as the **Shen (Spirit Influence)** for this system, representing **unconventional wisdom, adaptability, and the ability to see beyond illusion**.

Understanding this system provides insight into **how we meet change, how we regulate stress, and how we cultivate resilience** in the face of uncertainty. The tables below summarize its key attributes:

Zhen ☳ (Thunder) – The Spark of Change

Zhen ☳ (Thunder)	Details
Element	Wood
Direction	East
Attributes	Activation, initiation, movement, boldness, resilience
Feng Shui Associations	The Eldest Son, force of change, awakening, courage in the face of uncertainty - Activate Movement & Flow – Open pathways in your space; remove obstacles to encourage dynamic energy. - Incorporate Wood & Rising Energy – Plants, vertical elements, and upward-growing structures stimulate resilience. - Symbolic Drums & Sound – Instruments or chimes can amplify the energy of initiation and transformation.
Feng Shui Considerations	- Lightning as Metaphor – Sharp, sudden bursts of insight or change should be embraced rather than resisted.

Yang Wei Mai (Yang Linking Vessel) – The Web of Readiness

Yang Wei Mai (Yang Linking Vessel)	Immune & Response System
Function	Links all Yang channels, organizing the body's immune response, stress adaptation, and movement readiness. - The Yang Wei Mai is the body's first response to stimulus—the quickening, the surge of readiness. - It determines how we react to stress, challenge, and external demands.
Lineage – The First Shock of Awakening	- Before birth, it prepares the nervous and immune systems to meet the world, ensuring adaptability and resilience. - In fascia, the Yang Wei Mai corresponds to elasticity and rapid recoil, ensuring quick mobilization and dynamic protection. - It determines how we engage with change, how we take action, and how we set boundaries.
Belonging – The Web of Readiness	- A strong Yang Wei Mai allows for quick, dynamic engagement, while imbalance may lead to hyper-vigilance, exhaustion, or rigidity. - The Yang Wei Mai teaches movement, decision-making, and the art of stepping forward. - It is the line of warriors, performers, and those who act with immediacy.
Teaching Line – The Line of Boldness & Action	- Its lessons are learned through challenge, through movement, and through the willingness to leap.

Zhang Guolao (張果老) – The Mystic Alchemist

Zhang Guolao	Shen
Role	Patron of longevity, Daoist magic, and innovation.
	- Known as an eccentric hermit and master of Daoist magic.
	- Said to have lived in the Tang Dynasty, but legends claim he was hundreds of years old.
Cultural Significance	- Deeply respected by Tang emperors, who sought his wisdom, though he preferred solitude.
Symbol	Fish-Drum (鱼鼓, yúgǔ) – A drum used for summoning spirits and predicting the future.
	- He rode a white donkey backward, which could fold into a piece of paper when not in use.
Key Legend	- He refused royal invitations, claiming that worldly power was fleeting compared to the Dao.

Balance & Imbalance of the Zhen/Yang Wei Mai System

The **Zhen/Yang Wei Mai pairing** embodies **movement, resilience, and rapid adaptation**. When in balance, it allows for **quick, precise responses to stress and immune challenges**, maintaining a sense of **boldness and ease in action**.

However, **excess activation** can lead to **hyper-vigilance, burnout, or reactivity**, while **deficiency** results in **stagnation, lack of confidence, or weak immunity**. The body's ability to **respond to external forces without overreacting** is key to **both physical health and energetic vitality**.

By attuning to **Zhen's electric dynamism** and **Yang Wei Mai's web of readiness**, we learn to **engage with change, take decisive action, and trust in life's unfolding rhythms**.

Zhen ☳ / Yang Wei Mai State	Effects
	- Hyper-Vigilance & Overreaction – Jumping at every stimulus, feeling the need to "fix" or intervene constantly. - Adrenal Fatigue & Burnout – The body is in constant readiness, leading to exhaustion and depletion.
Excess (Overactive State)	- Rigidity in Beliefs & Actions – Holding onto control instead of adapting, resisting new perspectives. - Inability to Take Initiative – Feeling stuck, lacking momentum to move forward. - Fear of Change & Uncertainty – Over-identifying with past structures, resisting transformation.
Deficiency (Weakened State)	- Weak Boundaries & Lack of Direction – Struggling with assertion, being easily swayed by external forces. - Fluid Yet Focused – Able to respond with precision, neither hesitating nor overreacting. - Initiating with Awareness – Engaging in movement and decision-making without fear or rigidity.
Balanced State (Ideal Expression)	- Trust in the Unfolding Path – Seeing the rhythm of change as a natural flow.

Applying the Zhen/Yang Wei Mai Pairing in Practice

Influence	Details
	- Riding Backwards as a Perspective Shift – Seeing things from a different angle rather than reacting impulsively. - The Drumbeat of Change – Life has a rhythm; knowing when to act decisively versus when to pause and listen is key.
Afferent (Perception) – Zhang Guolao's Shen Influence	- Longevity through Adaptability – Resistance to change exhausts energy, while flexibility allows longevity. - Fast-Twitch Readiness – The ability to respond rather than react, maintaining awareness in movement. - Courage to Engage – Developing embodied confidence through action rather than avoidance.
Efferent (Action) – Yang Wei Mai's Structural Expression	- Training the Response System – Cultivating resilience in uncertainty by strengthening the body's capacity to adapt.

Xun ☴ (Wind) – The Belt Vessel & The Noble Patron

In the framework of **Neuroaffective Somatics**, each trigram from the **Bagua (八卦)** is mapped to an **Extraordinary Vessel**, which governs deep **physiological and energetic regulation**. The trigram **Xun ☴ (Wind)** corresponds to the **Dai Mai (Belt Vessel)**, the body's **only horizontal vessel**, responsible for **structural coherence, circulation, and energetic boundaries**.

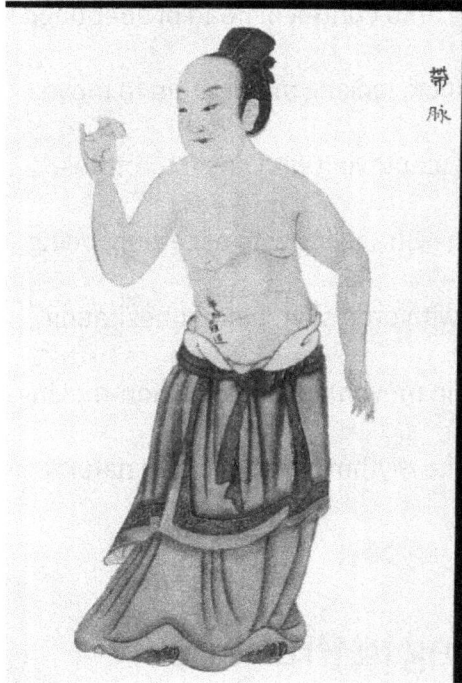

This pairing is associated with **balance, adaptability, and inheritance**, reflected in **how the body circulates blood and Qi, integrates ancestral patterns, and maintains structural integrity**. The legendary Taoist **Immortal Cao Guojiu** serves as the **Shen (Spirit Influence)** for this system, representing **justice, discipline, and mastery over inherited structures**.

Understanding this system provides insight into **how we hold structure, how we circulate energy, and how we refine our personal and ancestral legacies**. The tables below summarize its key attributes:

Xun ☴ (Wind) – The Breath of Circulation

Xun ☴ (Wind)	Details
Element	Wood
Direction	Southeast
Attributes	Flexibility, expansion, wisdom, structural balance, inheritance
Feng Shui Associations	Eldest daughter, lineage, strategy, planning, adjusting to forces beyond control - Encourage Airflow & Circulation – Open windows, use flowing fabrics, and avoid clutter to allow Qi to move freely. - Incorporate Wood & Flexible Structures – Bookshelves, wooden furniture, and organic shapes support adaptability. - Honor Legacy & Wisdom – Display heirlooms, meaningful texts, or symbols of discipline and justice.
Feng Shui Considerations	- Balance Containment & Flow – Use decorative elements that define space without restricting movement (e.g., room dividers rather than solid walls).

Dai Mai (Belt Vessel) – The Axis of Integration

Dai Mai (Belt Vessel)	Circulatory & Structural System
Function	Encircles the body, stabilizing **Qi circulation, core stability, and energetic coherence.** - The **Dai Mai** is the only **horizontal vessel**, acting as a **belt that holds vertical structures together.** - In **utero**, it forms the **axis of containment**, shaping **how the body stores and integrates inherited patterns.**
Lineage – The Binding Thread of Inheritance	- It determines how we **"hold" ancestral influences**—whether we **carry them fluidly or rigidly.** - The Dai Mai is the **fascia of containment**, regulating **core stability, postural integrity, and emotional boundaries.** - It influences **how we hold tension, whether we can digest experience, and how we define personal space.**
Belonging – The Vessel of Integration & Boundaries	- A **strong Dai Mai** provides **a sense of internal structure,** while **imbalance** can lead to **feeling fragmented, uncentered, or overly bound by the past.** - The **Dai Mai teaches the balance** between **holding and releasing, containment and flow.**
Teaching Line – The Line of Structural Wisdom	- It is the line of **choreographers, architects, and those who balance structure with movement.** - Its lessons are learned through **alignment—knowing when to hold and when to let go.**

Cao Guojiu (曹國舅) – The Noble Patron

Cao Guojiu	Shen
Role	Patron of justice, discipline, and noble virtue. - A Song Dynasty nobleman who abandoned his privileged life to pursue enlightenment.
Cultural Significance	- Symbolizes law, order, and self-discipline in Daoist thought.
Symbol	Jade Tablet – Represents authority, wisdom, and spiritual leadership. - After seeing the corruption of his family, he left to seek spiritual truth and became an Immortal.
Key Legend	- He embodies the balance of structure and transcendence.

Balance & Imbalance of the Xun/Dai Mai System

The **Xun/Dai Mai pairing** embodies **circulation, structural integrity, and the ability to hold or release inherited patterns**. When in balance, it allows for **smooth blood and Qi flow, clear emotional boundaries, and an ability to honor the past without being bound by it**.

However, **too much containment** can lead to **rigidity, fixation, or restriction**, while **too little structure** results in **instability, lack of direction, or weak energetic boundaries**. The body's ability to **hold structure without being trapped in it** is essential for **both circulatory health and personal sovereignty**.

By attuning to **Xun's flexible intelligence** and **Dai Mai's integrative containment**, we learn to **circulate energy wisely, set clear boundaries, and balance tradition with transformation**.

Xun ☴ / Dai Mai State	Effects
	- Over-Control & Rigidity – Holding onto ancestral or personal expectations too tightly.
	- Fixation on Rules & Hierarchy – Using structure to dominate rather than support flexibility.
Excess (Overactive State)	- Tension in the Core & Diaphragm – The body holds too much, restricting breath and movement.
	- Lack of Boundaries – Difficulty defining personal space, emotional limits, or self-discipline.
	- Feeling Fragmented or Unstable – Energy leaks, lack of coherence between upper and lower body.
Deficiency (Weakened State)	- Postural Collapse & Digestive Imbalance – Weakness in core stability, poor digestion of both food and experiences.
	- Firm Yet Flexible – Clear personal boundaries without rigidity.
	- Strategic Yet Adaptable – The ability to adjust to change while maintaining core integrity.
Balanced State (Ideal Expression)	- Justice in Action – Holding structure where needed, releasing where necessary.

Applying the Xun/Dai Mai Pairing in Practice

Influence	Details
	- Refinement of Lineage – Deciding what ancestral wisdom to keep and what to release.
	- Authority Over Self – Learning discipline without rigidity, maintaining inner sovereignty.
Afferent (Perception) – Cao Guojiu's Shen Influence	- Justice as an Internal Principle – Understanding fairness and self-regulation before imposing control externally.
	- Integration of Inherited Patterns – Holding stability in the core, releasing tension from past conditioning.
	- Movement Without Restriction – Learning when to contain and when to let go.
Efferent (Action) – Dai Mai's Structural Expression	- Architectural Awareness – Seeing the body as a structured yet adaptable system.

Li ☲ (Fire) – The Penetrating Vessel & The General-Healer

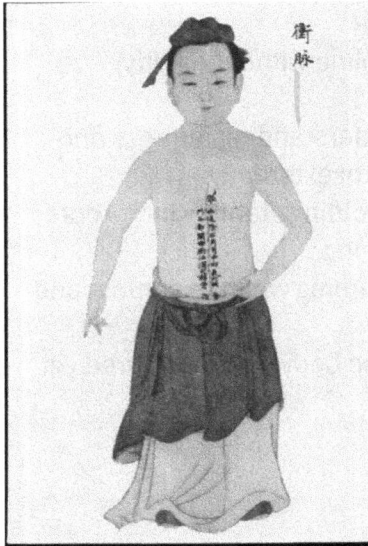

In the framework of **Neuroaffective Somatics**, each trigram from the **Bagua (八卦)** is mapped to an **Extraordinary Vessel**, which governs deep **physiological and energetic regulation**. The trigram **Li ☲ (Fire)** corresponds to the **Chong Mai (Penetrating Vessel)**, the body's **core channel for digestion, blood flow, and ancestral imprinting**.

This pairing is associated with **transformation, illumination, and deep integration**, reflected in **how the digestive system processes nutrients, how the blood carries ancestral imprints, and how we metabolize both food and experience**. The legendary Taoist **Immortal Zhongli Quan** serves as the **Shen (Spirit Influence)** for this system, representing **alchemy, healing, and the ability to transmute old wounds into wisdom**.

Understanding this system provides insight into **how we assimilate nourishment, how we transform inherited patterns, and how we embody deep ancestral intelligence**. The tables below summarize its key attributes:

Li ☲ (Fire) – The Furnace of Transformation

Li ☲ (Fire)	Details
Element	Fire
Direction	South
Attributes	Illumination, transformation, wisdom, passion, ancestral memory
Feng Shui Associations	The Sun, radiance, inner fire, vision, deep alchemical shifts
Feng Shui Considerations	- Enhance Warmth & Circulation – Use warm lighting, candles, and elements that promote movement of energy. - Incorporate Fire & Transformation Symbols – Red, triangular shapes, and representations of transmutation (alchemy, Phoenix imagery, sacred fires). - Balance Heat & Flow – If the space feels stagnant, add movement (e.g., water features to cool excess fire, mirrors to reflect light) without dampening passion. - Objects of Power & Wisdom – Display symbols of healing, ancestral strength, and transformation.

Chong Mai (Penetrating Vessel) – The River of Assimilation

Chong Mai (Penetrating Vessel)	
Function	**Digestive & Circulatory System** Regulates digestion, blood flow, and deep ancestral memory, harmonizing the processing of nutrients, emotions, and inherited patterns. - The Chong Mai is the deepest vessel, carrying the imprint of generational energy, emotions, and life force. - It is the original vessel of embryonic circulation, linking us to the bloodlines of our ancestors.
Lineage – The Blood River of Ancestry	- It holds the charge of inherited traumas, strengths, and core identity formation, affecting digestion, blood quality, and emotional processing. - In fascia, the Chong Mai corresponds to the midline core and deep front line, influencing posture, circulation, and gut health. - It governs how we metabolize core emotions, how we process intensity, and how we embody personal identity.
Belonging – The Vessel of Deep Memory & Identity	- A well-regulated Chong Mai allows for deep connection to self, while imbalance can lead to feeling lost in generational patterns or overwhelmed by deep emotions. - The Chong Mai teaches how to work with what we inherit—how to transform old patterns into something new. - It is the line of alchemists, therapists, and those who engage in deep ancestral work.
Teaching Line – The Line of Ancestral Power & Transformation	- Its lessons are learned through introspection, facing deep emotional currents, and conscious transformation of inherited patterns.

Zhongli Quan (鐘離權) – The General-Healer

Zhongli Quan	Shen
Role	Patron of medicine, healing, and spiritual transformation.
Cultural Significance	- A former Han Dynasty general, who after losing a battle, retreated to the mountains and was initiated into Daoist alchemy and healing. - Often depicted as a fat, jovial sage, symbolizing abundance and wisdom.
Symbol	Fan – Represents healing and the ability to revive the dead.
Key Legend	- Discovered a secret text on alchemy, granting him knowledge of the Dao. - Trained Lü Dongbin and tested him with ten temptations before accepting him as a disciple.

Balance & Imbalance of the Li/Chong Mai System

The **Li/Chong Mai pairing** governs **digestion, emotional integration, and transformation**. When in balance, it fosters **strong digestion, clear emotional processing, and the ability to metabolize both food and experience efficiently**.

However, **too much fire** can lead to **inflammation, burnout, or emotional overwhelm**, while **too little fire** results in **poor circulation, sluggish digestion, and lack of passion**. The body must be able to **digest what it receives—whether it's food, emotions, or ancestral inheritance—without being consumed by it**.

By attuning to **Li's illuminating energy** and **Chong Mai's deep currents**, we learn to **process what nourishes us, release what does not, and transmute past experiences into wisdom**.

Li ☲ / Chong Mai

State	Effects
	- Over-Identification with Past Trauma – Feeling stuck in generational wounds, unable to move forward.
	- Burnout & Overexertion – The fire burns too hot, leading to fatigue, anxiety, or inflammatory conditions.
Excess (Overactive State)	- Emotional Flooding – Too much energy surging at once, overwhelming the system.
	- Lack of Connection to Roots – Feeling disconnected from lineage, identity, or deep wisdom.
	- Poor Circulation & Stagnation – Blood, Qi, and emotions become blocked, leading to stiffness or coldness in body or spirit.
Deficiency (Weakened State)	- Loss of Passion or Direction – A dimmed fire, lack of vitality, or a sense of being lost.
	- Transformation as a Living Process – Engaging with change without fear or resistance.
	- Deep Presence & Ancestral Awareness – Feeling rooted yet expansive, supported but sovereign.
Balanced State (Ideal Expression)	- Fire as Power, Not Destruction – Using intensity for clarity, movement, and healing.

Applying the Li/Chong Mai Pairing in Practice

Influence	Details
	- From Wound to Wisdom – How personal and ancestral wounds can be transformed into medicine.
	- Holding & Releasing – Recognizing that not all inheritance must be carried forward.
Afferent (Perception) – Zhongli Quan's Shen Influence	- Alchemy of Identity – The ability to reshape self-concept through awareness and practice.
	- Deep Circulatory Intelligence – Regulating how life force moves through the body.
	- Integration of Emotional Currents – Learning to process rather than suppress intensity.
Efferent (Action) – Chong Mai's Structural Expression	- Embodied Transformation – Taking ancestral weight and transmuting it into strength.

Kan ☵ (Water) – The Yin Linking Vessel & The Androgynous Wanderer

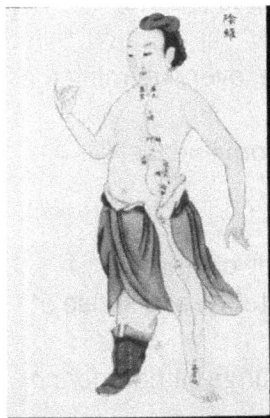

In the framework of **Neuroaffective Somatics**, each trigram from the **Bagua (八卦)** is mapped to an **Extraordinary Vessel**, which governs deep **physiological and energetic regulation**. The trigram **Kan ☵ (Water)** corresponds to the **Yin Wei Mai (Yin Linking Vessel)**, the body's **network of emotional containment, connective tissue stability, and adaptive fluidity**.

This pairing is associated with **depth, surrender, and emotional intelligence**, reflected in **how fascia interweaves through the body, how emotions are metabolized, and how we cultivate inner stability amidst constant change**. The legendary Taoist **Immortal Lan Caihe** serves as the **Shen (Spirit Influence)** for this system, representing **impermanence, detachment, and the fluidity of identity**.

Understanding this system provides insight into **how we hold and release emotions, how we navigate change, and how we embody the wisdom of impermanence**. The tables below summarize its key attributes:

Note: The art in this section is from **WikiCommons**.

Kan ☵ (Water) – The Depths of Reflection

Kan ☵ (Water)	Details
Element	Water
Direction	North
Attributes	Depth, emotion, reflection, adaptability, surrender
Feng Shui Associations	The Middle Son, the abyss, mystery, hidden wisdom, the unconscious mind
	- Encourage Flow & Depth – Introduce water features, mirrors, or curved pathways to reflect emotional movement.
	- Incorporate Symbols of Impermanence – Art that represents cycles, fluidity, or transient beauty.
	- Create a Restorative Space – Use soft blues, deep purples, and organic textures that invite introspection.
Feng Shui Considerations	- Balance Light & Dark – Kan represents the deep unknown—consider mood lighting or spaces for stillness and meditation.

Yin Wei Mai (Yin Linking Vessel) – The Web of Emotional Containment

Yin Wei Mai (Yin Linking Vessel) **Function**	Fascia & Emotional Processing System Links all Yin channels, harmonizing internal energy, emotional resilience, and connective tissue integrity. - The Yin Wei Mai holds the emotional signatures of our lineage, regulating how we process and express emotions. - It connects how past experiences shape our inner world, carrying the emotional memory of our ancestors.
Lineage – The Vessel of Emotional Inheritance	- It is the bridge between past pain and present healing, determining how we metabolize deep emotional experiences. - The Yin Wei Mai is the fascia of emotional containment, influencing how we digest, metabolize, and integrate deep emotions. - It governs how we feel safe within our own emotions, how we connect to inner stillness, and how we create stability in shifting emotional landscapes.
Belonging – The Vessel of Emotional Processing & Inner Stability	- A strong Yin Wei Mai allows for deep emotional wisdom, while imbalance may lead to emotional flooding, repression, or difficulty trusting one's feelings. - The Yin Wei Mai teaches us how to hold and integrate emotion, how to find wisdom in what we feel.
Teaching Line – The Line of Deep Reflection & Emotional Mastery	- It is the line of philosophers, contemplatives, and those who master emotional intelligence. - Its lessons are learned through deep reflection, stillness, and harmonizing past experiences with present awareness.

Lan Caihe (藍采和) – The Androgynous Wanderer

Lan Caihe	Shen
Role	Patron of minstrels, beggars, and free spirits; embodies spontaneity and detachment from material wealth.
	- Described as androgynous, eccentric, and unpredictable. - Wore ragged clothes and often sang cryptic Daoist poems about impermanence and illusion.
Cultural Significance	- Associated with street performers and the disenfranchised, emphasizing non-attachment and creative freedom.
Symbol	Flower Basket – Represents impermanence, beauty, and artistic expression.
	- One day, Lan Caihe vanished into the clouds, leaving behind only a tattered robe. - Often depicted giving away riches, emphasizing detachment from material
Key Legend	wealth.

Balance & Imbalance of the Kan/Yin Wei Mai System

The **Kan/Yin Wei Mai pairing** governs **emotional integration, adaptability, and the resilience of the connective tissue system**. When in balance, it fosters **fluid emotional processing, deep wisdom, and a stable yet adaptable body structure**.

However, **excess emotional containment** can lead to **stagnation, attachment to suffering, or rigidity**, while **too little containment** results in **emotional flooding, instability, or avoidance of depth**. The ability to **hold and release experience without grasping or resisting** is essential for **both emotional and physical resilience**.

By attuning to **Kan's deep reflective nature** and **Yin Wei Mai's stabilizing fascia**, we learn to **surrender to change, process emotions with wisdom, and cultivate adaptability without losing our center**.

Kan ☵ / Yin Wei Mai State	Effects
	- Overwhelm & Emotional Flooding – Feeling drowned by emotions, unable to process them fully. - Hyper-Sensitivity & Disconnection – Swinging between deep feeling and emotional numbness.
Excess (Overactive State)	- Attachment to Suffering – Identifying too much with pain or loss, unable to release old wounds. - Avoidance of Emotion – Struggling to sit with discomfort or process grief. - Lack of Emotional Depth – Feeling shallow, unfulfilled, or emotionally disconnected.
Deficiency (Weakened State)	- Fear of Letting Go – Holding onto relationships, beliefs, or emotions that need release. - Fluid & Adaptable – Able to move through emotions with ease, neither clinging nor avoiding. - Emotionally Wise & Centered – Finding depth in stillness, trusting the ebb and flow of life.
Balanced State (Ideal Expression)	- Creative & Free-Spirited – Embracing life's uncertainties as opportunities for growth.

Applying the Kan/Yin Wei Mai Pairing in Practice

Influence	Details
	- Seeing Beauty in Change – Recognizing the impermanence of both suffering and joy. - Detachment from Material Expectation – Learning to release what no longer serves.
Afferent (Perception) – Lan Caihe's Shen Influence	- The Fluidity of Identity – Understanding that who we are is ever-evolving. - Emotional Processing & Containment – The ability to hold deep emotions without being overwhelmed. - Softness as Strength – Practicing emotional resilience through surrender, not resistance.
Efferent (Action) – Yin Wei Mai's Structural Expression	- Inner Stability in Uncertain Waters – Remaining centered amidst shifting tides.

Dui ☱ (Lake) – The Yang Heel Vessel & The Daoist Musician

In the framework of **Neuroaffective Somatics**, each trigram from the **Bagua (八卦)** is mapped to an **Extraordinary Vessel**, which governs deep **physiological and energetic regulation**. The trigram **Dui ☱ (Lake)** corresponds to the **Yang Qiao Mai (Yang Heel Vessel)**, the body's **network of externalized action, physical confidence, and energy distribution**—closely linked to the **endocrine system's role in regulating stress, vitality, and expression**.

This pairing is associated with **joy, spontaneity, and resonance**, reflected in **how the endocrine system modulates energy levels, how movement expresses presence, and how we cultivate confidence in action**. The legendary Taoist **Immortal Han Xiangzi** serves as the **Shen (Spirit Influence)** for this system, representing **music, vibrational healing, and the freedom of creative expression**.

Understanding this system provides insight into **how we balance action and rest, how we assert our presence, and how we attune to the rhythms of expression and engagement**. The tables below summarize its key attributes:

Dui ☱ (Lake) – The Flow of Joyful Expression

Dui ☱ (Lake)	Details
Element	Metal
Direction	West
Attributes	Joy, expression, refinement, harmony, spontaneity
Feng Shui Associations	The Youngest Daughter, music, movement, artistic creativity, the power of voice
	- Encourage Expression & Creativity – Open areas for movement, music, or artistic engagement.
	- Incorporate Metal Elements – Bells, chimes, or reflective surfaces enhance clarity and resonance.
	- Balance Sound & Silence – Create spaces for both vibrancy and rest, ensuring harmony in daily rhythms.
Feng Shui Considerations	- Symbolic Flute or Wind Instruments – Representing breath, voice, and effortless flow in movement.

Yang Qiao Mai (Yang Heel Vessel) – The Pulse of Dynamic Engagement

Yang Qiao Mai (Yang Heel Vessel)	Endocrine & Energy Regulation System
Function	Governs **externalized action, physical readiness, and energy distribution**, balancing **dynamic expression and stillness**.
	- The **Yang Qiao Mai** regulates how we **move outward**, how we **claim space**, and how we **interact with the external world**.
	- It determines how we **embody confidence, forward movement, and self-projection**.
	- It is the vessel of **assertion, readiness, and momentum**, directly
Lineage – The Vessel of Externalized Action	influencing **hormonal responses to stress, excitement, and performance**.
	- In **fascia**, the Yang Qiao Mai corresponds to the **outer fascial chains**, governing **how we move dynamically through space**.
	- It influences **confidence, facial expression, and how we step forward with strength**.
Belonging – The Vessel of Motion & Engagement	- A **strong Yang Qiao Mai** allows for a **clear presence**, while imbalance can lead to **hesitation, difficulty asserting oneself, or excessive aggression**.
	- The **Yang Qiao Mai teaches** confidence, courage, and the ability to **take up space without fear**.
	- It is the line of **leaders, performers, and those who step forward**
Teaching Line – The Line of Leadership & Direction	with clarity.
	- Its lessons are learned through **motion, presence, and the willingness to fully inhabit one's space**.

Han Xiangzi (韓湘子) – The Daoist Musician

Han Xiangzi	Shen
Role	Patron of musicians, poets, and harmony.
	- Nephew of Confucian scholar Han Yu, but rejected Confucian ideals in favor of Daoist mysticism and music.
Cultural Significance	- Known for his ability to make flowers bloom instantly and communicate with nature through music.
Symbol	Flute – Represents music's power to harmonize the universe.
	- Angered his Confucian uncle by rejecting strict logic in favor of Daoist spontaneity.
	- His **flute could control wind and water**, symbolizing **the power of sound as a vibrational force**.
Key Legend	

Balance & Imbalance of the Dui/Yang Qiao Mai System

The **Dui/Yang Qiao Mai pairing** governs **expression, physical confidence, and the regulation of energy levels through the endocrine system**. When in balance, it allows for **effortless movement, clear expression, and dynamic presence**.

However, **too much externalization** can lead to **overperformance, restlessness, or burnout**, while **too little expression** results in **hesitation, blocked creativity, or fear of being seen**. The ability to **move with clarity, assert without force, and express with ease** is essential for **hormonal and energetic balance**. By attuning to **Dui's joyfulness** and **Yang Qiao Mai's energetic rhythms**, we learn to **express ourselves authentically, engage dynamically, and embody confidence without strain**.

Dui ☱ / Yang Qiao Mai State	Effects
	- Over-Performance & Burnout – Constantly "on," needing validation through action.
	- Restlessness & Overextension – Difficulty pausing, feeling the need to always be in motion.
Excess (Overactive State)	- Overbearing Presence – Speaking or acting without tuning into the environment.
	- Hesitation & Insecurity – Holding back, struggling to occupy space with confidence.
Deficiency (Weakened State)	- Blocked Expression – Feeling stifled creatively or socially.
	- Fear of Visibility – Difficulty being seen, heard, or fully present.
	- Embodied Presence – Moving with clarity, rhythm, and grace.
	- Authentic Expression – Feeling safe to speak, create, and engage without self-doubt.
Balanced State (Ideal Expression)	- Joyful Resonance – Living in tune with oneself and the surrounding world.

Applying the Dui/Yang Qiao Mai Pairing in Practice

Influence	Details
	- Music as Medicine – Recognizing vibration and resonance as tools for healing and connection. - Spontaneity & Freedom – The ability to move with life rather than against it.
Afferent (Perception) – Han Xiangzi's Shen Influence	- Authentic Self-Expression – Trusting one's own voice and presence. - Dynamic Embodiment – Stepping into physical confidence and movement. - Harmony in Motion – Finding ease and grace in expression, rather than forcing outcomes.
Efferent (Action) – Yang Qiao Mai's Structural Expression	- Energetic Projection – Learning to balance external action with internal awareness.

Gen ☶ (Mountain) – The Yin Heel Vessel & The Iron-Crutch Wanderer

In the framework of **Neuroaffective Somatics**, each trigram from the **Bagua (八卦)** is mapped to an **Extraordinary Vessel**, which governs deep **physiological and energetic regulation**. The trigram **Gen ☶ (Mountain)** corresponds to the **Yin Qiao Mai (Yin Heel Vessel)**, the body's **primary system for rest, deep recovery, and respiratory balance**.

This pairing is associated with **stillness, endurance, and deep vision**, reflected in **how the respiratory system regulates breath cycles, how the body shifts between rest and activity, and how we integrate subconscious awareness into waking life**. The legendary Taoist **Immortal Li Tieguai** serves as the **Shen (Spirit Influence)** for this system, representing **resilience through suffering, transcendence, and hidden wisdom**.

Understanding this system provides insight into **how we regulate breath, how we access deep rest, and how stillness itself becomes a source of power**. The tables below summarize its key attributes:

Note: The art in this section is from **WikiCommons**.

Gen ☶ (Mountain) – The Depth of Stillness

Gen ☶ (Mountain)	Details
Element	Earth
Direction	Northeast
Attributes	Stillness, vision, restoration, endurance, depth
Feng Shui Associations	The Youngest Son, deep knowing, rest, slowness, the hidden inner world - Create Stillness & Grounding – Design spaces for meditation, contemplation, and deep rest. - Incorporate Earth Elements – Stones, clay, and heavy, grounding materials to support stability. - Honor the Unseen – Use subtle lighting, hidden alcoves, or objects representing deep wisdom.
Feng Shui Considerations	- Symbolic Crutches or Walking Sticks – Representing support, resilience, and the wisdom of limitation.

Yin Qiao Mai (Yin Heel Vessel) – The Breath of Restoration

Yin Qiao Mai (Yin Heel Vessel)	Respiratory & Restorative System
Function	Regulates respiratory rhythms, sleep cycles, and deep subconscious healing, balancing activity and rest.
	- The Yin Qiao Mai governs rest, introspection, and the ability to turn inward.
	- Before birth, it establishes the rhythms of sleep, deep cellular restoration, and parasympathetic regulation.
Lineage – The Vessel of Deep Stillness	- It is the vessel of pause, stillness, and inner reflection, directly influencing the lungs' ability to regulate breath and oxygenation during sleep and meditation.
	- The Yin Qiao Mai regulates the slow, deep networks of structural support, governing our ability to rest and recover.
	- It shapes how we experience deep relaxation, sleep cycles, and subconscious processing.
Belonging – The Vessel of Restoration & Dreaming	- A well-regulated Yin Qiao Mai allows for deep embodiment and restful awareness, while imbalance may lead to insomnia, chronic tension, or dissociation.
	- The Yin Qiao Mai teaches the power of stillness, reflection, and moving from deep internal knowing.
	- It is the line of poets, dreamers, and those who access deep vision through rest and introspection.
Teaching Line – The Line of Dreaming & Visionary Depth	- Its lessons are learned through silence, through the unseen, and through the ability to trust what is felt rather than what is seen.

Li Tieguai (李鐵拐) – The Iron-Crutch Wanderer

Li Tieguai	Shen
Role	Patron of the sick, the poor, and Daoist mysticism.
	- Depicted as a crippled beggar with a gourd, symbolizing humility and resilience.
Cultural Significance	- Though physically disabled, he possessed great spiritual power and helped the suffering.
Symbol	Iron Crutch & Gourd – Represents immortality, medicine, and transcendence over suffering.
	- He accidentally lost his original body, so his soul took over the corpse of a lame beggar.
Key Legend	- Despite his rough appearance, he had deep wisdom and compassion.

Balance & Imbalance of the Gen/Yin Qiao Mai System

The **Gen/Yin Qiao Mai pairing** governs **restorative breathing, deep sleep cycles, and the integration of subconscious wisdom**. When in balance, it allows for **calm, steady breath, deep restful sleep, and the ability to slow down without fear of stagnation**.

However, **too much stillness** can lead to **stagnation, isolation, or difficulty engaging with life**, while **too little stillness**results in **restlessness, chronic stress, and disrupted breathing patterns**. The ability to **pause, restore, and trust in stillness** is essential for **both respiratory health and mental clarity**.

By attuning to **Gen's deep quietude** and **Yin Qiao Mai's restorative cycles**, we learn to **breathe fully, rest deeply, and access the wisdom held in stillness**.

Gen ☶ / Yin Qiao Mai State	Effects
	- Stagnation & Isolation – Withdrawing too much, losing touch with external reality.
	- Fear of Engagement – Choosing inertia over action, staying trapped in past wounds.
Excess (Overactive State)	- Insomnia & Nervous Tension – Struggling to fully surrender to rest and recovery.
	- Restlessness & Burnout – Inability to pause, feeling driven by constant motion.
	- Lack of Inner Awareness – Difficulty accessing deep self-knowledge or trusting intuition.
Deficiency (Weakened State)	- Disconnection from the Body – Feeling ungrounded, adrift, or dissociated.
	- Embodied Stillness – Feeling rested and present in both mind and body.
	- Wisdom Through Experience – Integrating life's lessons without being trapped by suffering.
Balanced State (Ideal Expression)	- Deep Vision & Intuition – Trusting one's inner knowing and ability to move at the right time.

Applying the Gen/Yin Qiao Mai Pairing in Practice

Influence	Details
	- Embracing Limits as Strength – Recognizing that disability or restriction can refine inner power. - Seeing Beyond Appearances – Understanding wisdom is not in form but in presence.
Afferent (Perception) – Li Tieguai's Shen Influence	- Resilience Through Stillness – Learning that depth arises when we stop forcing movement. - Rest as Restoration – Understanding pause is not weakness, but power. - Dreaming as Healing – Working with subconscious processing and inner vision.
Efferent (Action) – Yin Qiao Mai's Structural Expression	- Balancing Movement & Stillness – Learning when to act and when to be still.

#	System	Vessel	Trigram	Element	Immortal	Functions
1	Nervous System	Du Mai (Governing Vessel)	☰ Qian (Heaven)	Metal	Lü Dongbin (Scholar-Sage)	Spinal integrity, nervous system regulation, inherited strength, structural willpower
2	Reproductive System	Ren Mai (Conception Vessel)	☷ Kun (Earth)	Earth	He Xiangu (Immortal Maiden)	Gestation, hormonal balance, fertility, Yin receptivity, maternal lineage
3	Immune System	Yang Wei Mai (Yang Linking Vessel)	☳ Zhen (Thunder)	Wood	Zhang Guolao (Mystic Alchemist)	Defense, rapid response, adaptability, boundary-setting, resilience
4	Circulatory System	Chong Mai (Penetrating Vessel)	☲ Li (Fire)	Fire	Zhongli Quan (General-Turned-Healer)	Blood flow, cardiovascular regulation, ancestral memory, transformation
5	Digestive System	Dai Mai (Belt Vessel)	☴ Xun (Wind)	Wood	Cao Guojiu (Noble Patron)	Core stability, digestion, processing nourishment, integration of experience
6	Connective Tissue	Yin Wei Mai (Yin Linking Vessel)	☵ Kan (Water)	Water	Lan Caihe (Androgynous Wanderer)	Fascial memory, emotional holding, deep adaptability, somatic inheritance
7	Endocrine System	Yang Qiao Mai (Yang Heel Vessel)	☱ Dui (Lake)	Metal	Han Xiangzi (Daoist Musician)	Hormonal rhythms, metabolic cycles, external engagement, self-expression
8	Respiratory System	Yin Qiao Mai (Yin Heel Vessel)	☶ Gen (Mountain)	Earth	Li Tieguai (Iron-Crutch Wanderer)	Breathing cycles, deep rest, parasympathetic tone, stillness and recovery

Contemplations for the Eight Extraordinary Vessels

☰ Qian (Heaven) – The Pure Potential of Motion

- Where do I feel the upward movement of energy in my body? How does it change with breath or posture?
- How do I experience alignment between vision, purpose, and movement?
- What does "Heaven" feel like in my practice—expansive, guiding, distant?

☷ Kun (Earth) – The Ground of Being

- Where do I feel most stable in my body? Where do I resist grounding?
- How does my connection to the ground shift when I surrender vs. when I brace?
- What happens when I move from deep stability rather than force?

☳ Zhen (Thunder) – The Sudden Spark of Energy

- How does my body react to sudden shifts—do I brace, flow, or expand?
- What is my first instinct when energy surges—containment or release?
- Where in my body do I feel "Thunder"—as sensation, impulse, or tension?

☴ Xun (Wind) – Flowing With and Through

- What is my relationship to control and surrender in movement?
- Where do I allow flow vs. where do I create unnecessary resistance?
- How do I recognize the difference between force and attunement?

☲ Li (Fire) – Illumination & Expression

- Where does movement originate in my body when I feel inspired?
- What happens when I allow my body to express energy without hesitation?
- What movement feels like "fire"—expansive, rising, consuming, transformative?

☵ Kan (Water) – Depth & Adaptation

- How do I experience fluidity in movement vs. rigidity?
- Where in my body do I hold emotional depth—what movements unlock it?
- What changes when I allow movement to be effortless, like water finding its own path?

☱ Dui (Lake) – Reflection & Internal Resonance

- What sensations arise when I slow down and listen inwardly?
- How do I respond when movement becomes more about sensing than doing?
- What emerges when I let stillness be part of movement?

☶ Gen (Mountain) – The Weight of Presence

- How does stillness feel in my body—stable, tense, or grounding?
- Where do I feel the greatest resistance to pausing and waiting?
- What happens when I move from deep presence rather than reaction?

Postures

The following pages contain information for approximately 30 postures that have been placed in the following groups; Transitions, Head Neck and Shoulders, Backbends, Hips and Pelvis, and Twists/Side Body

I've given you an image, some essential instructions, benefits, and ways to customize. Contemplate these as ingredients in recipes you create. Any timing I share is, of course, merely a suggestion.

For my Fellow Hypermobile Humans:

We benefit more from doing less, so please be curious about how deep you go and how long you hold these postures.

You will note that not all postures have information on the meridians – this is most often true in transition postures, such as Savasana. For these deeply relaxing moments, the aim is towards homeostasis, so the meridians, while present, aren't necessarily being 'worked'. Your mileage may vary, of course

Please also note that these categories are somewhat arbitrary and that many postures fit into more than one category and, therefore, can be used in more than one way.

"Activating" Meridians

If you are stretching, and you are aware of it, **all** of your body is involved. "Activating" has to do with the direction that our tissues are being expanded towards. If the shape expands the heart meridian, I shared it as active.

A different resource might have different information, and that is OK. Contemplating singular shapes is a fully modern moment ☺ .

Sequences

I've included some suggestions for combinations at the end of this section. Please use them as recipes and not prescriptions

Transitions

Transitions: Creating Flow Between Postures

Transitions help the body shift smoothly between postures, allowing for a sense of continuity and integration. These movements are not just in-between moments; they provide an opportunity for the nervous system to adjust, the breath to deepen, and the body to prepare for what comes next.

Some transitions, like **Savasana**, offer a moment of stillness between more active poses, while others, like **Happy Baby**, can help unwind tension before moving into a new focus area. Whether used to reset, release, or prepare, transitions are an essential part of a balanced practice.

The Transitions covered here include:

- Constructive Rest Position
- Table Top
- Cat/Cow
- Child's Pose
- Happy Baby
- Hugging the Earth
- Legs Up the Wall
- Savasana

Constructive Rest Position (Hatha)

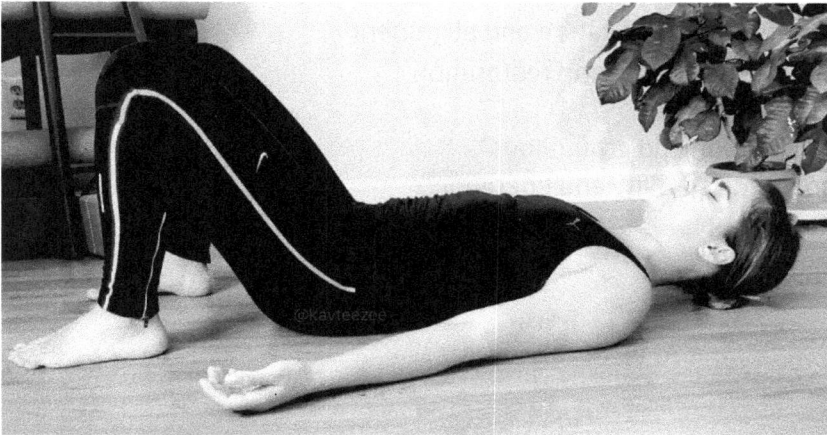

Instructions

1. Lie on your back with your knees bent and feet flat on the floor.
2. Keep your feet hip-width apart and positioned under your knees.
3. Allow your spine to rest in its natural shape—avoid pressing it into the floor or over-arching.
4. Relax your arms by your sides, palms facing up or down.
5. Breathe deeply and remain in the position for 5–20 minutes.

Effects

✔ Gently releases tension in the psoas muscle
✔ Supports spinal decompression and natural alignment
✔ Encourages diaphragmatic breathing and relaxation
✔ Helps counteract "tech neck" and poor posture

Considerations

! Low back sensitivity—some may feel discomfort without support
! Knee strain—adjust foot positioning if needed
! Neck discomfort—head positioning may need modification

Customizations

◆ Place a small roll under the low back to encourage a neutral spine
◆ Let the knees rest together for additional relaxation
◆ Elevate the feet on a chair for added support

Meridian	Element	Function in Pose
Bladder	Water (Yang)	Supports spinal relaxation and alignment
Kidney	Water (Yin)	Facilitates deep rest and restoration
Stomach	Earth (Yang)	Aids digestion and grounding
Spleen	Earth (Yin)	Encourages stability and energetic nourishment

Table Top

Instructions

1. Begin on all fours with your hands stacked directly under your shoulders and knees under your hips.
2. Keep your spine neutral, avoiding excessive arching or rounding.
3. Distribute weight evenly through your hands and knees.
4. Engage your core and lengthen through the crown of your head.
5. Hold for several breaths or use as a transition into other movements.

Effects

✓ Establishes a neutral spine
✓ Prepares the body for movement and transitions
✓ Engages core stability and weight distribution

Considerations

! Wrist pain or sensitivity
! Knee discomfort
! Foot or ankle pain

Customizations

◆ Make fists with the hands for wrist sensitivity
◆ Pad the knees with a blanket for added comfort
◆ Tuck the toes or place the tops of the feet down based on preference

Meridian Alignments

Meridian	Element	Function in Pose
Bladder	Water (Yang)	Supports spinal relaxation and alignment
Kidney	Water (Yin)	Facilitates deep rest and restoration
Stomach	Earth (Yang)	Aids digestion and grounding
Spleen	Earth (Yin)	Encourages stability and energetic nourishment

Hugging the Earth (Self-Awakening)

A grounding pose that releases tension in the neck and shoulders while promoting deep relaxation.

Instructions

1. Lie down on your belly with your arms extended forward.
2. Turn your head to one side, resting your cheek on the mat.
3. Slightly tuck your chin to release tension in the neck.
4. Relax your jaw and let your entire body soften into the ground.
5. Hold for 2–3 minutes per side, then switch.

Effects

✔ Grounds the anterior line of the body
✔ Encourages a deep sense of relaxation
✔ Gently stretches the neck and upper back

Considerations

! Pregnancy
! Lower back pain
! Knee or ankle discomfort

Customizations

◆ Place a blanket or towel under the forehead for support
◆ Bend the knees slightly to ease pressure on the lower back
◆ Rest the forehead on stacked hands instead of turning the head

Meridian Alignments

Meridian	Element	Function in Pose
Stomach (胃)	Earth (Yang)	Grounds energy and aids digestion
Spleen (脾)	Earth (Yin)	Supports nourishment and emotional grounding
Lung (肺)	Metal (Yin)	Encourages breath awareness and relaxation
Large Intestine (大肠)	Metal (Yang)	Supports release and letting go

Cat/Cow, Fluid Cat/Cow

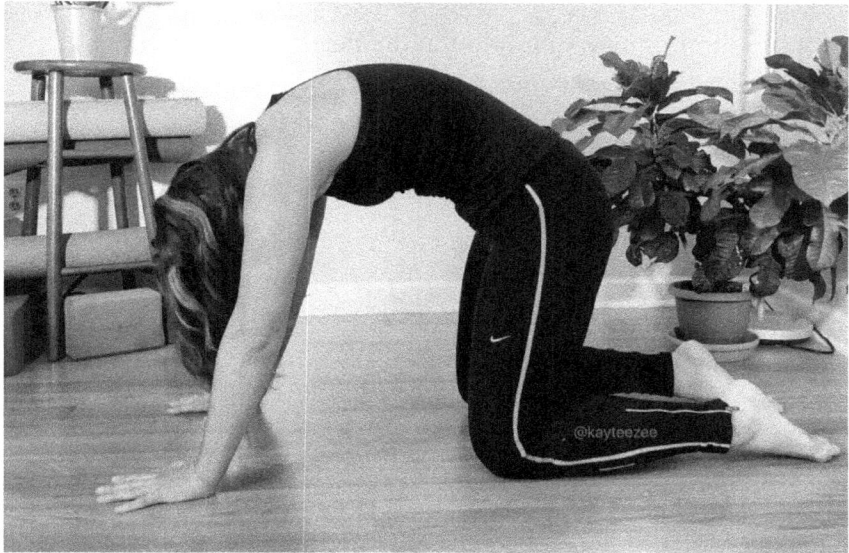

A foundational movement sequence that mobilizes the spine, enhances breath awareness, and promotes spinal flexibility.

Instructions

1. Begin in **Tabletop Position**, with hands under shoulders and knees under hips.
2. **Exhale**: Press your hands into the floor, round your back, and tuck your chin toward your chest, feeling a stretch across your spine (**Cat Pose**).
3. **Inhale**: Drop your belly, lift your chest and chin, and gently arch your back (**Cow Pose**).
4. Repeat this movement in sync with your breath for several rounds.
5. **For Fluid Cat-Cow**: Move intuitively, adding circular or wave-like motions as needed.

Effects

✓ Stretches and mobilizes the spine

✓ Enhances coordination of breath and movement

✓ Encourages spinal movement in six directions

Considerations

! Neck pain or injury—limit range of motion in the head

! Wrist sensitivity—adjust hand placement or use fists

! Foot or knee discomfort—modify with props for support

Customizations

◆ Make fists with the hands to reduce wrist strain

◆ Place a blanket under the knees for added comfort

◆ Keep the head neutral if experiencing neck sensitivity

Meridian Alignment

Meridian	Element	Function in Pose
Bladder (膀胱)	Water (Yang)	Supports spinal flexibility and movement
Kidney (肾)	Water (Yin)	Nourishes deep energy reserves
Stomach (胃)	Earth (Yang)	Stimulates digestion and core activation
Spleen (脾)	Earth (Yin)	Enhances grounding and fluid motion

Childs Pose

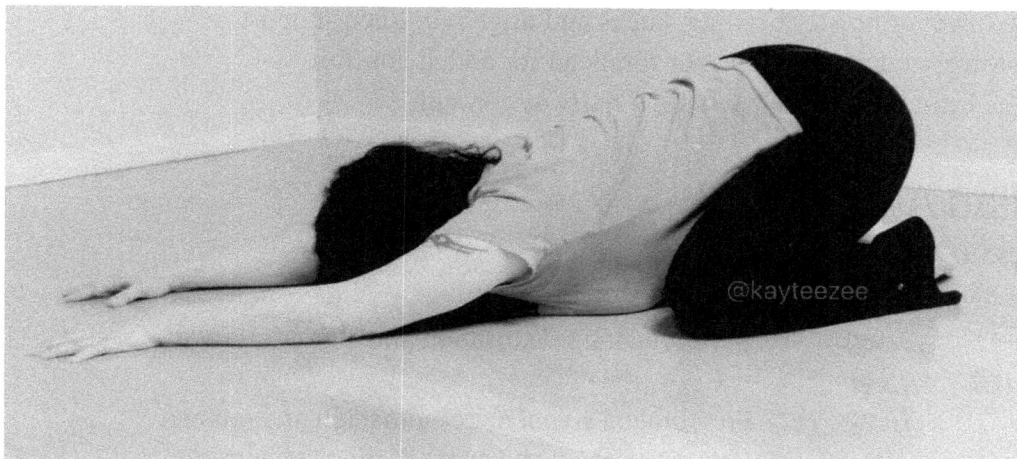

A grounding and restorative posture that calms the nervous system and gently stretches the spine, hips, and shoulders.

Instructions

1. Begin in **Tabletop Position** or seated on your heels.
2. Bring your **big toes to touch** and **sit back onto your heels**, allowing your knees to open wide.
3. Extend your **arms forward**, resting your forehead on the floor.
4. Relax your shoulders and breathe deeply into your back and hips.
5. Hold for **2-3 minutes** or longer for deeper relaxation.

Effects

✓ Calms the nervous system and turns senses inward
✓ Gently stretches the spine, hips, and shoulders
✓ Encourages deep diaphragmatic breathing

Considerations

! Pregnancy—keep knees wider and avoid deep compression
! Shoulder or neck pain—adjust arm placement for comfort
! Knee or foot sensitivity—use props for support

Customizations

◆ Move the torso toward one leg to stretch the opposite side body
◆ Place a towel or bolster between knees and thighs for knee support
◆ Rest a towel under feet, knees, or forehead for added comfort
◆ Turn the head to one side, switching halfway through

Meridian Alignment

Meridian	Element	Function in Pose
Kidney (肾)	Water (Yang)	Supports deep restoration and energy storage
Bladder (膀胱)	Water (Yang)	Encourages spinal decompression and release
Stomach (胃)	Earth (Yang)	Grounds energy and soothes the digestive system
Spleen (脾)	Earth (Yin)	Promotes nourishment and energetic stability

Happy Baby

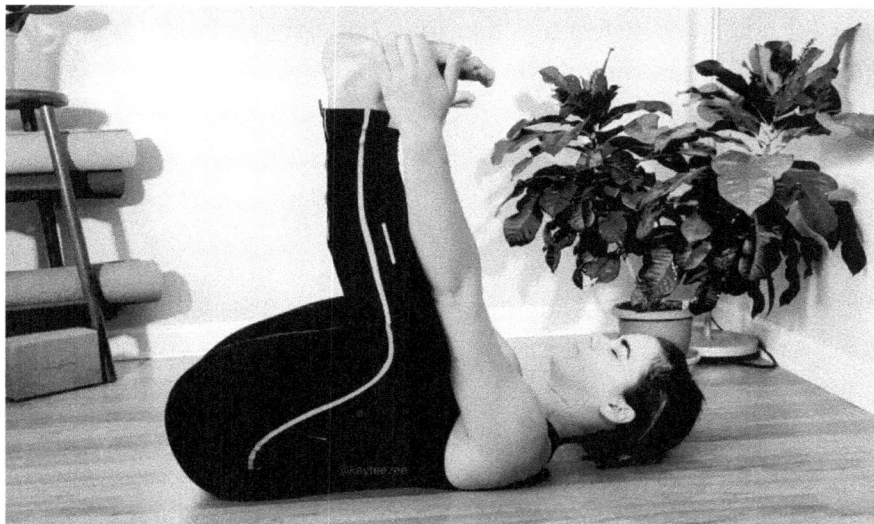

A gentle hip opener that decompresses the spine while stretching the inner thighs, hamstrings, and lower back.

Instructions

1. **Lie on your back** with your knees bent and feet lifted toward the ceiling.
2. Keep your **knees at a 90-degree angle** and align them over your hips.
3. Reach for the **outer edges of your feet** (or ankles/shins if needed).
4. Gently pull your knees down toward your armpits while keeping your spine flat.
5. Hold for **up to 3 minutes**, breathing deeply.

Effects

✓ Flattens and decompresses the spine
✓ Deep groin and hip stretch
✓ Stretches hamstrings and inner thighs

Considerations

! Low back curvature—ensure the spine remains grounded
! Groin or SI joint sensitivity—ease into the pose slowly
! Knee or ankle discomfort—modify with hand placement

Customizations

◆ **Half Happy Baby** – Extend one leg while keeping the other bent
◆ **Feet Together** – Press soles of feet together for a butterfly variation
◆ **Hold Behind Knees** – If reaching the feet strains the back

Meridian Alignment

Meridian	Element	Function in Pose
Bladder (膀胱)	Water (Yang)	Encourages spinal decompression and fluid movement
Kidney (肾)	Water (Yin)	Supports deep relaxation and flexibility
Liver (肝)	Wood (Yin)	Promotes emotional release and flow
Gallbladder (胆)	Wood (Yang)	Stimulates lateral movement and decision-making energy
Heart (心)	Fire (Yin)	Encourages openness and circulation in the chest
Small Intestine (小肠)	Fire (Yang)	Enhances spinal alignment and energetic clarity

Legs Up the Wall

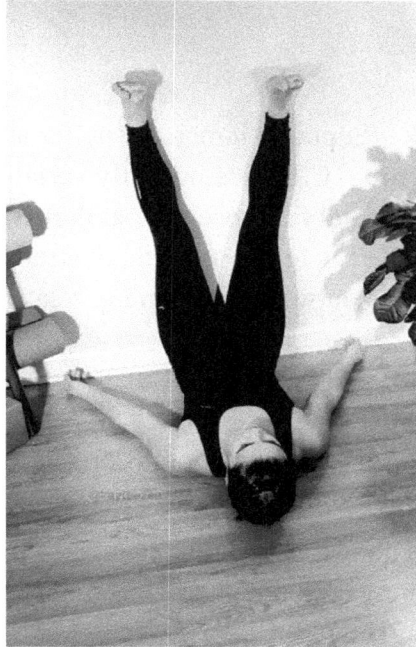

A restorative inversion that promotes circulation, reduces swelling, and calms the nervous system.

Instructions

1. Sit with your **hip close to the wall**, then lie onto your back and extend your legs up the wall.
2. Adjust your **hips slightly away** if needed for comfort.
3. Let your **arms rest comfortably** by your sides or on your abdomen.
4. Keep your **neck neutral**, ensuring it's not strained forward or back.
5. Expand through your **upper back**, allowing full relaxation.
6. Hold for **5-10 minutes**, breathing deeply.

Effects

✓ Encourages circulation and reduces **edema in legs and feet**
✓ Supports **lymphatic drainage** and venous return
✓ **Calms the nervous system**, promoting relaxation

Considerations

! **Glaucoma** – Inversions may increase eye pressure
! **Numbness in legs** – Adjust or bring soles together if needed
! **Neck discomfort** – Ensure proper support for alignment

Customizations

◆ **Towel/Bolster Under Lower Back** – Supports lumbar spine for added comfort
◆ **Soles Together, Heels Toward Groin** – Creates a butterfly variation for hip release
◆ **Support the Head** – Especially beneficial for those with **arthritis or neck tension**
◆ **Straddle Against the Wall** – Widens legs for an inner thigh stretch
◆ **Frog Against the Wall** – Bends knees outward for deep hip relaxation

Meridian Alignment

Meridian	Element	Function in Pose
Bladder (膀胱)	Water (Yang)	Encourages spinal decompression and relaxation
Kidney (肾)	Water (Yin)	Supports deep rest and fluid balance
Spleen (脾)	Earth (Yin)	Aids in circulation and fluid movement
Stomach (胃)	Earth (Yang)	Helps with digestion and grounding energy
Heart (心)	Fire (Yin)	Regulates circulation and emotional calmness

Savasana – Corpse Pose

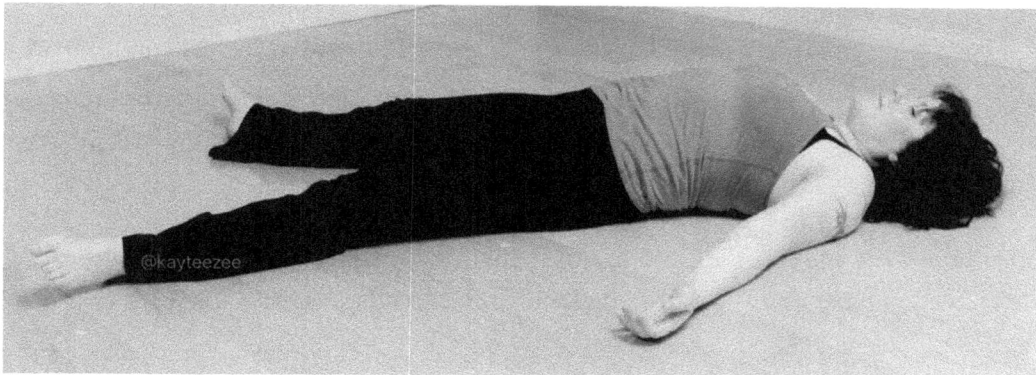

A deep relaxation posture that allows full integration of movement, breath, and stillness.

Instructions

1. Lie down on your **back**, allowing your arms and legs to rest naturally.
2. Keep your **feet slightly apart**, letting them fall open.
3. Turn your **palms upward** to encourage openness and relaxation.
4. Allow your **breath to settle**, moving effortlessly in and out.
5. Hold for **5-20 minutes**, releasing any remaining tension.
6. To exit, **roll to one side**, pause, and gently press up to a seated position.

Effects

✓ Encourages **nervous system regulation** and deep relaxation
✓ **Resets postural patterns**, allowing the spine to settle in **neutral alignment**
✓ Acts as the **threshold between practice and daily life**, integrating movement and stillness

Considerations

! **Neck pain** – Support the head and adjust positioning for comfort
! **Low back pain** – Modify with props to reduce discomfort

Customizations

◆ **Blanket/Towel Under Head** – Supports cervical alignment and relaxation
◆ **Bolster Under Knees** – Reduces strain on the lower back and promotes spinal decompression
◆ **Towel Under Low Back/Sacrum** – Helps some people find greater ease
◆ **Knees Bent into Constructive Rest** – Provides additional low back support

Meridian Mapping

Meridian	Element	Function in Pose
Bladder (膀胱)	Water (Yang)	Facilitates spinal relaxation and nervous system reset
Kidney (肾)	Water (Yin)	Supports deep rest, restoration, and energy storage
Pericardium (心包)	Fire (Yin)	Helps release emotional tension and cultivates inner peace
Stomach (胃)	Earth (Yang)	Encourages digestive ease and grounding energy
Spleen (脾)	Earth (Yin)	Nourishes and stabilizes the body during deep rest

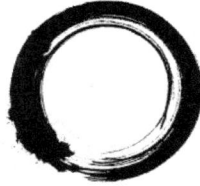

Head, Neck, and Shoulders

Many Yin Yoga practices primarily focus on the **ribcage to the knees**, emphasizing deep stretches in the hips and lower body. While this is valuable, **connective tissue exists throughout the body**, and neglecting the upper body can leave areas of chronic tension unaddressed.

If you spend time on your phone or work at a desk—like most people today—you're likely familiar with **"smartphone neck"** and **shoulder stiffness**. Prolonged sitting, screen time, and repetitive motions create **tension patterns in the neck, shoulders, and upper back** that Yin Yoga can help release.

By incorporating **postures that target the upper body**, you can restore balance, relieve tension, and support **full-body mobility**. These additions create a more **rounded practice**, helping you move and feel better—both on and off the mat.

The postures for the Head Neck and Shoulders included here are:

Seated Neck Stretch

Thread the Needle

Shoulder Pigeon

Hand Stretch

Seated Neck Stretch (Forrest)

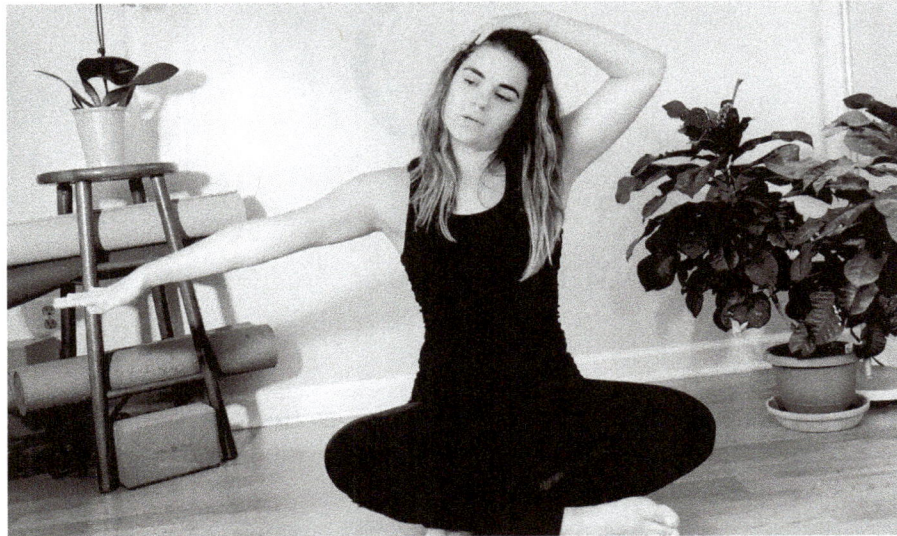

Seated Neck Stretch

A simple yet effective stretch to release tension in the **neck, shoulders, and jaw**.

Instructions

1. **Sit cross-legged** or in a comfortable seated position.
2. Let your **left ear fall toward your left shoulder**, keeping both shoulders relaxed.
3. Extend your **right arm outward**, about a foot off the ground, to deepen the stretch.
4. For added intensity, **gently place your left hand on the right side of your head**, allowing the natural weight of your arm to enhance the stretch.
5. Hold for **up to 2 minutes**, breathing deeply into the side of your neck.
6. Use your **left hand/arm to guide your head back to center**.
7. Switch the cross of your legs and **repeat on the opposite side**.

Effects

✔ Stretches the **scalene, trapezius, and sternocleidomastoid** muscles
✔ Can relieve **TMJ discomfort** and jaw tension
✔ Helps alleviate **tension headaches**
✔ Encourages **shoulder relaxation and postural awareness**

Considerations

! Be mindful of **pinched nerves**—if you feel tingling or sharp pain, ease out of the stretch
! **Less is more**—modulate the intensity rather than forcing the movement

Customizations

◆ **Reduce intensity** by keeping your supporting hand off your head
◆ **Adjust the chin angle** slightly to target different areas of the neck
◆ **Keep hands resting on the lap** for a gentler version
◆ If sitting cross-legged is uncomfortable, **sit on a chair or elevate hips** on a cushion

Meridian Alignment

Meridian	Element	Function in Pose
Small Intestine (小肠)	Fire (Yang)	Supports clarity, relaxation, and posture awareness
Large Intestine (大肠)	Metal (Yang)	Encourages release of tension and energetic flow
Lungs (肺)	Metal (Yin)	Aids breath expansion and emotional release

Thread the Needle

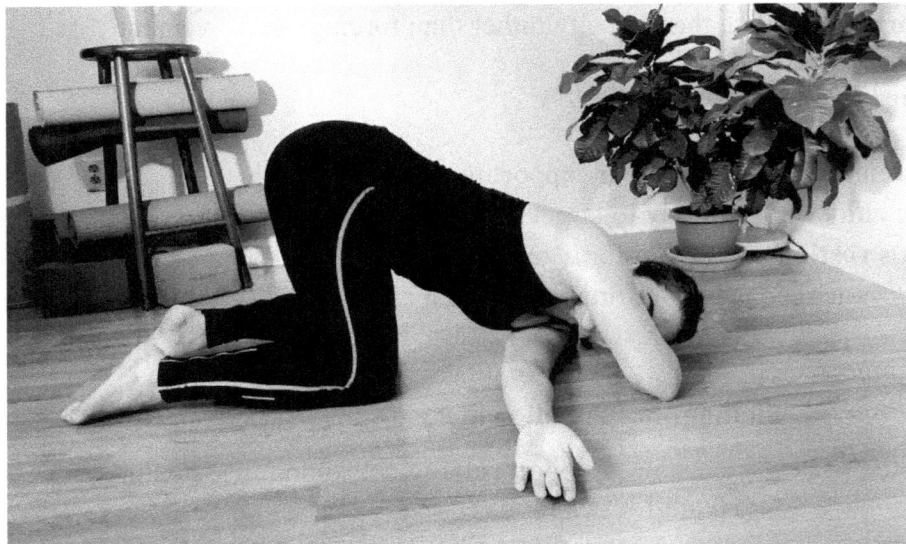

A **gentle spinal twist** that releases **tension in the upper back, shoulders, and neck** while promoting relaxation.

Instructions

1. Start in **Tabletop Position** (hands under shoulders, knees under hips).
2. **Inhale**, then **thread your right arm under your left**, bringing your right shoulder and temple to the floor.
3. Allow your **left hand to support you** or extend it forward for a deeper stretch.
4. Keep your **hips level** and breathe deeply into the upper back.
5. Hold for **1–2 minutes**, softening with each exhale.
6. **Slowly return** to Tabletop and **repeat on the other side**.

Effects

✓ Stretches **upper back, shoulders, and side body**
✓ Encourages **spinal rotation and release of tension**
✓ Supports **deep, diaphragmatic breathing**

Considerations

⚠ Avoid if experiencing **neck pain, disc herniation, or severe shoulder tightness**
⚠ For **knee discomfort**, use padding under the knees

Customizations

◆ Place a **blanket under knees or head** for support
◆ Extend the **opposite leg back** for a full-body stretch (right arm threads, extend left leg)
◆ Wrap the **free arm behind the back** for a deeper shoulder opening
◆ Lift the **same-side leg** as the free arm for added balance and core engagement

Meridian Alignment

Meridian	Element	Function in Pose
Small Intestine (小肠)	Fire (Yang)	Opens the back and shoulders, aiding clarity and relaxation
Large Intestine (大肠)	Metal (Yang)	Encourages release of stored tension, aids circulation
Triple Warmer (三焦)	Fire (Yang)	Regulates nervous system balance and overall body flow

Shoulder Pigeon

A **deep anterior shoulder opener** that also engages the **chest, upper back, and thoracic spine** through gentle rotation.

Instructions

1. **Lie prone** on your belly with your legs extended.
2. Extend your **right arm perpendicular** to your torso, palm facing down.
3. **Slowly roll onto your right side**, using your **left foot as a rudder** to guide the movement.
4. Keep your **right shoulder grounded** and breathe into the stretch.
5. Hold for **3–4 minutes**, softening with each exhale.
6. **Gently return** to the belly before switching sides.

Effects

✓ Opens the **anterior shoulder, chest, and upper arm**
✓ Releases **tension in the thoracic spine**
✓ Encourages **heart-centered awareness**

Considerations

⚠ Avoid if experiencing **rotator cuff injuries, shoulder impingement, or wrist pain**
⚠ Modify if there is **AC joint sensitivity or discomfort in the neck**

Customizations

◆ Keep the **arm extended** without rolling back for a gentler variation
◆ Use a **block or towel under the head** for neck support
◆ Adjust the **leg placement** to control intensity—fully rolling onto the side deepens the stretch

Meridian Alignment

Meridian	Element	Function in Pose
Heart (心, Xīn)	Fire (Yin)	Expands the chest, encourages emotional release
Small Intestine (小肠, Xiǎocháng)	Fire (Yang)	Facilitates connection between the arms, shoulders, and heart
Pericardium (心包, Xīnbāo)	Fire (Yin)	Protects the heart, regulates circulation, and relieves emotional tension

Hand Stretch

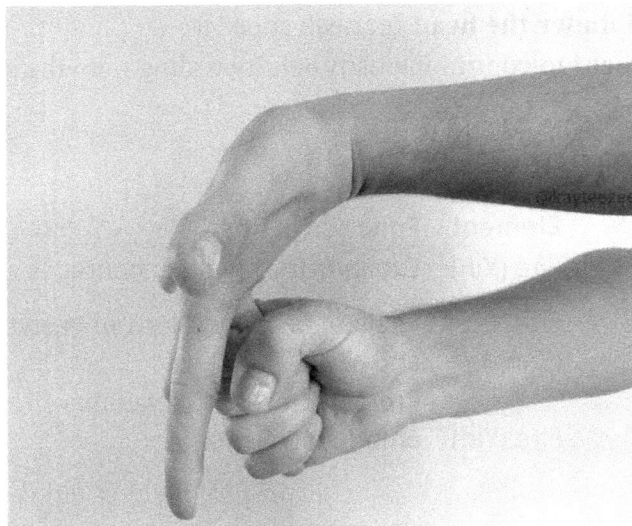

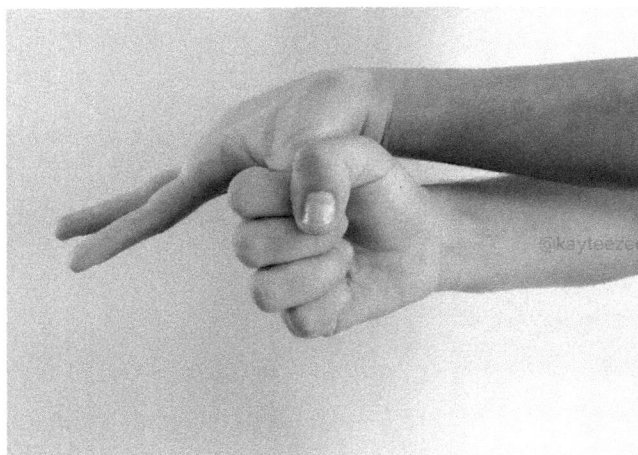

A **gentle yet effective stretch** that increases **flexibility in the fingers, hands, and wrists**, promoting circulation and **relieving tension from repetitive movements.**

Instructions

1. **Extend your right hand forward**, spreading your fingers wide.
2. **Grip your pinky finger** with your left hand and gently pull it back.
3. **Repeat for each finger**, moving from pinky to index.
4. For the **thumb**, place the backs of your hands together first, then gently pull back.
5. Hold each stretch for **several breaths**, keeping the rest of the hand relaxed.
6. Repeat on the **other hand.**

Effects

✓ **Increases mobility** in the hands, fingers, and wrists
✓ **Stretches the carpal tunnel** and **supports joint flexibility**
✓ **Relieves tension** from excessive grip use, typing, or repetitive hand movements

Considerations

⚠ Avoid excessive force if experiencing **arthritis, tendonitis, or recent hand injuries**
⚠ Modify for **carpal tunnel syndrome** by reducing stretch intensity

Customizations

◆ Perform a **lighter stretch** by pulling fingers back less aggressively
◆ **Massage the palms** or apply gentle pressure to acupressure points for added release
◆ **Support the wrist with the opposite hand** if experiencing sensitivity

Meridian Alignment

Meridian	Element	Function in Pose
Pericardium (心包, Xīnbāo)	Fire (Yin)	Opens circulation to the hands, relieves wrist strain
Triple Warmer (三焦, Sānjiāo)	Fire (Yang)	Balances movement between fingers, wrists, and forearms
Small Intestine (小肠, Xiǎocháng)	Fire (Yang)	Improves coordination between hand and shoulder
Heart (心, Xīn)	Fire (Yin)	Enhances finger dexterity and supports fine motor function
Lung (肺, Fèi)	Metal (Yin)	Supports breath awareness in hand movements
Large Intestine (大肠, Dàcháng)	Metal (Yang)	Clears tension and stiffness from the arms and shoulders

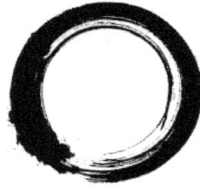

Backbends

Back pain is something that most adults experience at some point in life, and often back bending can alleviate some of that pain. Protector of the central nervous system, the spine plays a critical role in everything we do. In a Yin Yoga context, backbends remedy forward-facing actions and habits, such as sitting at a desk, driving, etc..

The Backbends included here are:

Puppy Pose

Sphinx Pose

Seal Pose

Supported Bridge

Puppy Pose

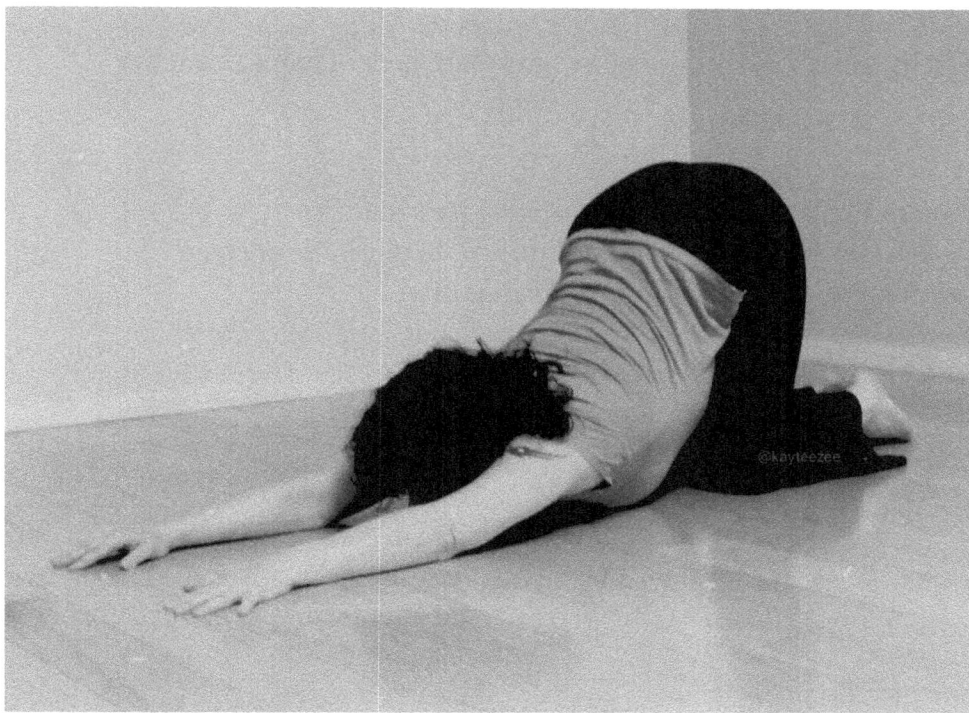

A **deep chest-opening posture** that **stretches the spine, shoulders, and heart center** while gently reversing forward-head posture.

Instructions

1. Begin in **Tabletop Position** (hands under shoulders, knees under hips).
2. **Walk your hands forward**, lowering your chest toward the ground.
3. Keep **hips stacked over the knees** and **arms extended forward**, palms down.
4. Rest your **chin or forehead on the floor**, ensuring the neck stays comfortable.
5. Hold for **up to 5 minutes**, breathing deeply into the stretch.

Effects

✓ **Heart opener** – Expands the chest and stimulates the heart and lungs
✓ **Releases upper back tension** – Especially beneficial for those with "smartphone neck"
✓ **Gently stretches the shoulders and arms**
✓ **Encourages deep diaphragmatic breathing**

Considerations

! Neck sensitivity – If discomfort arises, rest the **forehead** instead of the chin
! Knee pain – Pad under the knees for extra support
! Numbness or tingling in arms – Adjust hand placement or reduce duration

Customizations

◆ **Turn the chin to one side**, switching halfway for symmetry
◆ **Prop the chest with a bolster** or folded blanket for a gentler opening
◆ **Place a cushion under the knees** for added comfort
◆ **Bend the elbows** and rest the forehead on the hands for a softer variation
◆ **Supported Fish Pose** can be a great alternative if deep shoulder flexion is not accessible

Meridian Alignment

Meridian	Element	Function in Pose
Heart (心, Xīn)	Fire (Yin)	Expands the chest, opens the emotional center
Lung (肺, Fèi)	Metal (Yang)	Supports breath awareness and upper body expansion
Triple Warmer (三焦, Sānjiāo)	Fire (Yang)	Stimulates circulation through the arms and hands
Pericardium (心包, Xīnbāo)	Fire (Yin)	Encourages relaxation and stress relief

Sphinx Pose

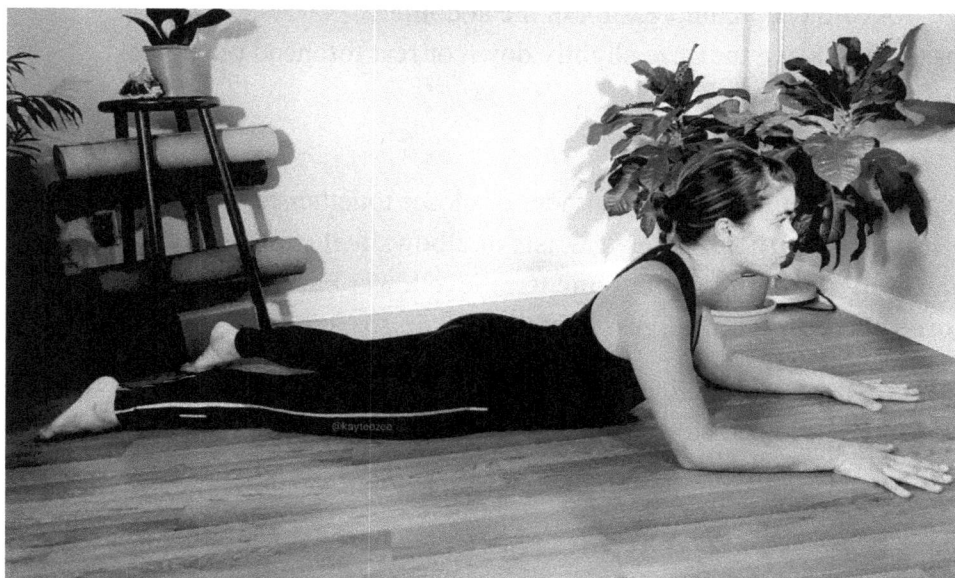

A gentle backbend that stimulates the lower spine, opens the chest, and encourages deep breathing.

Instructions

1. Begin **lying on your belly**, legs extended and relaxed.
2. Place **elbows under the shoulders** with **forearms parallel**, palms down.
3. Allow your **chest to soften forward** while the shoulders naturally lift.
4. Keep **lower body relaxed**, avoiding tension in the glutes or thighs.
5. **Tuck the chin slightly** or keep the neck neutral to avoid strain.
6. Hold for **up to 5 minutes**, breathing deeply into the lower back and abdomen.

Effects

✓ **Opens the lower back** – Stimulates lumbar and sacral arch
✓ **Encourages gentle spinal extension** without excessive compression
✓ **Expands the chest** – Supports deeper breath awareness
✓ **Supports digestion** by gently stimulating abdominal organs

Considerations

! Lower back pain – If discomfort arises, reduce intensity by moving elbows forward
! Pregnancy – Avoid deep compression in the abdomen
! Neck sensitivity – Keep the gaze slightly down or rest forehead on a block

Customizations

◆ **Adjust leg positioning** – Bring legs wider or closer together for comfort
◆ **Support forearms with a bolster** if wrists or elbows feel strained
◆ **Place a cushion above the pubic bone** to relieve lower back tension
◆ **For a more relaxed variation,** rest the forehead on stacked hands

Meridian Alignment

Meridian	Element	Function in Pose
Kidney (肾, Shèn)	Water (Yin)	Supports deep rest and grounding
Bladder (膀胱, Pángguāng)	Water (Yang)	Stimulates the spine and lumbar region
Stomach (胃, Wèi)	Earth (Yang)	Supports digestion and abdominal function
Spleen (脾, Pí)	Earth (Yin)	Encourages stability and nourishment
Liver (肝, Gān)	Wood (Yin)	Facilitates smooth Qi flow and detoxification
Gallbladder (胆, Dǎn)	Wood (Yang)	Aids in spinal mobility and decision-making

Seal Pose

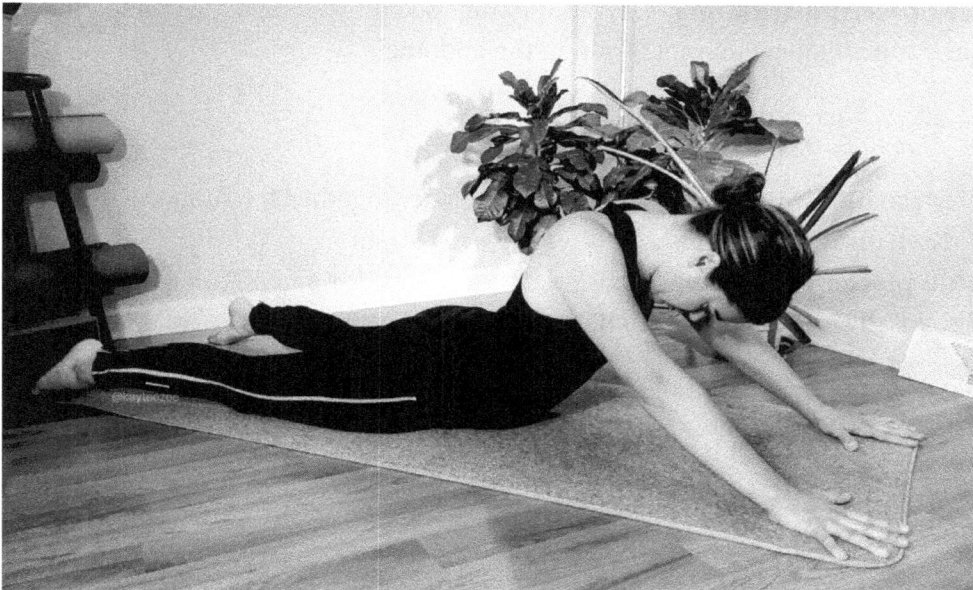

A **deep backbend** that **expands the chest, strengthens the spine, and stimulates the lower back.**

Instructions

1. **Begin in Sphinx Pose,** with **elbows under shoulders and forearms resting on the mat.**
2. **Straighten the arms,** lifting the chest higher while allowing the **shoulders to rise naturally.**
3. Keep **lower body relaxed,** avoiding unnecessary tension in the glutes or thighs.
4. Allow the **chest and heart to gently soften forward** to deepen the stretch.
5. Hold for **up to 5 minutes,** breathing into the **lumbar spine and lower ribs.**

Effects

✓ **Opens the lower back** – Creates space in the lumbar spine
✓ **Expands the chest and diaphragm** – Supports deeper breathing
✓ **Stimulates the sacral and lumbar region** – Enhances spinal mobility
✓ **Encourages abdominal organ function** – Aids digestion and circulation

Considerations

! **Lower back sensitivity** – If discomfort arises, lessen the arch or return to Sphinx
! **Shoulder or wrist discomfort** – Avoid locking the elbows and adjust hand placement
! **Pregnancy** – Avoid deep compression in the abdomen

Customizations

◆ **Adjust leg positioning** – Widen or bring legs closer together for support
◆ **Use a bolster under the forearms** to lessen wrist strain
◆ **Vary hand placement** – Bring hands slightly forward for a gentler backbend
◆ **Keep elbows slightly bent** if straightening the arms causes discomfort

Meridian Alignment

Meridian	Element	Function in Pose
Kidney (肾, Shèn)	Water (Yin)	Supports deep restoration and grounding
Bladder (膀胱, Pángguāng)	Water (Yang)	Stimulates spinal energy and fluid circulation
Stomach (胃, Wèi)	Earth (Yang)	Aids digestion and abdominal function
Spleen (脾, Pí)	Earth (Yin)	Provides stability and nourishment
Liver (肝, Gān)	Wood (Yin)	Facilitates smooth Qi flow and detoxification
Gallbladder (胆, Dǎn)	Wood (Yang)	Supports spinal mobility and emotional flexibility

Supported Bridge (Restorative)

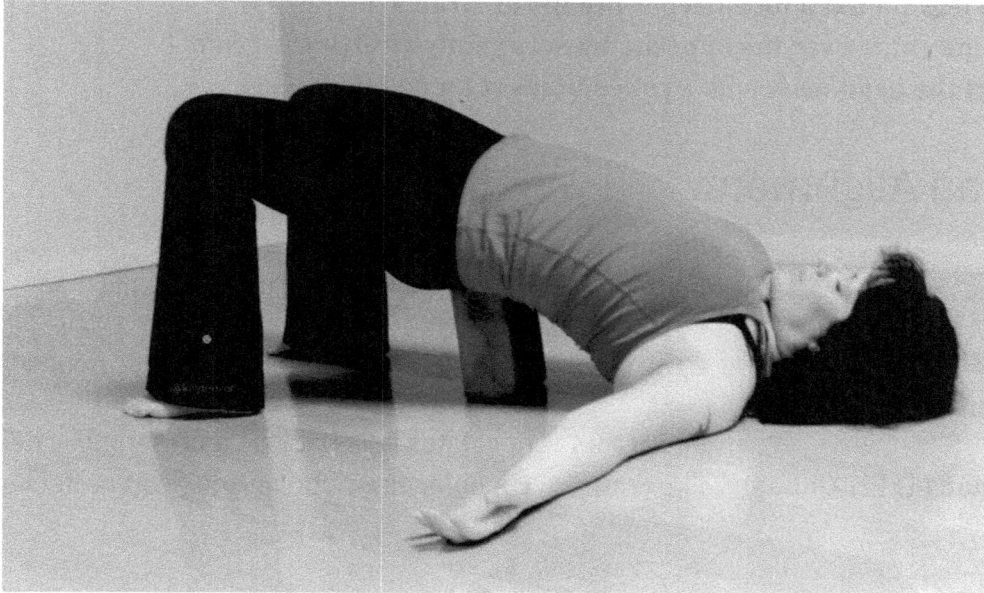

A **gentle backbend** that **supports spinal decompression, opens the hip flexors, and relieves lower back tension.**

Instructions

1. **Begin in Constructive Rest Position** – Lie on your back with **knees bent and feet hip-width apart.**
2. **Lift your hips** and place a **yoga block** or **bolster under your sacrum.**
3. **Relax into the support,** allowing your **spine to lengthen** and hips to settle.
4. Keep **arms relaxed,** with **palms facing up** or resting gently on the belly.
5. Hold for **up to 5 minutes,** breathing into the **abdomen and hip flexors.**

Effects

✓ **Decompresses the lower back** – Reduces spinal pressure and tension
✓ **Gently opens the hip flexors** – Encourages pelvic release
✓ **Stimulates circulation in the lower abdomen** – Supports digestive and reproductive health

Considerations

! **Sacral or lumbar pain** – Adjust block height or use a bolster for gentler support
! **Neck sensitivity** – Avoid overextending the neck; support with a blanket if needed
! **Pregnancy** – Modify by keeping the feet elevated

Customizations

◆ **Use a bolster instead of a block** for a **softer backbend**
◆ **Extend legs forward** for a **deeper hip flexor stretch**
◆ **Cross one ankle over the opposite knee** to **gently stretch the groin**
◆ **Support the head/neck** with a **rolled blanket** for additional ease

Meridian Alignment

Meridian	Element	Function in Pose
Stomach (胃, Wèi)	Earth (Yang)	Supports digestion and abdominal organ function
Spleen (脾, Pí)	Earth (Yin)	Provides grounding and energetic nourishment
Triple Warmer (三焦, Sānjiāo)	Fire (Yang)	Regulates fluid balance and metabolic heat
Pericardium (心包, Xīnbāo)	Fire (Yin)	Encourages emotional and heart protection

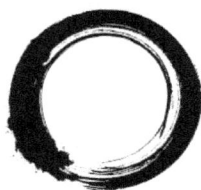

Hips and Pelvis

Hips: Gravity, Emotion & Connection

The **hips are the body's foundation**, deeply influenced by **gravity, movement, and stored emotions**. They are **the bridge between stability and mobility**, grounding us in **both structure and sensation**.

As some of the **largest joints** in the body, the hips are surrounded by **dense connective tissue and strong fascial lines**, making them a primary focus in **Yin Yoga and somatic practices**.

The **pelvis is the axis of transformation**—where **one becomes two** as the **spine splits into the legs**. It is the center of **balance, expression, and adaptability**, carrying the weight of **our history, emotions, and relationship with the ground**.

In many traditions, **the hips are considered a storage place for unprocessed experiences**, particularly **grief, fear, and tension**. Releasing the hips can unlock **deep-seated patterns**, restoring **ease and fluidity** in the whole body.

By **honoring gravity as an ally**, hip-opening postures invite a sense of **letting go**, allowing both **physical and emotional release** to arise with awareness.

The Hip postures included here are:

Butterfly	Shoelace
Double Pigeon	Toes Pose
Hero's Pose	
Dragon	Sleeping Swan
Caterpillar	

Butterfly Pose Seated/Folded

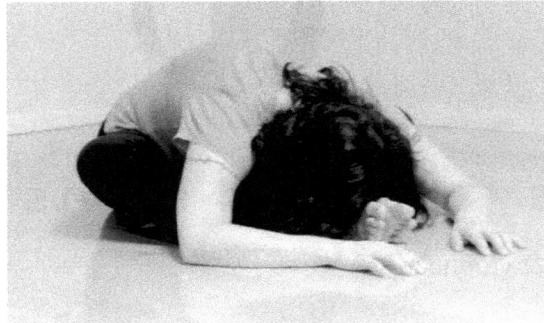

Instructions

1. Sit on the floor with the **soles of your feet together**, allowing your knees to open naturally.
2. Position your feet **about two feet from your groin** for a more accessible stretch.
3. **Gently fold forward**, rounding your spine and allowing your head to relax toward your feet.
4. Hold for **up to 5 minutes**, breathing deeply into your lower back and hips.

Effects

✓ **Deep groin stretch**
✓ **Opens inner thighs and hips**
✓ **Releases tension in the lower back**

Considerations

! **Groin strain or sensitivity**
! **SI joint discomfort**
! **Knee or ankle pain**

Customizations

◆ **Support your pelvis** by sitting on a block or folded blanket.
◆ **Place blocks or bolsters under your knees** if your hips feel tight.
◆ **Use a bolster for upper body support** if folding forward deeply.
◆ **Keep your spine long and chest lifted** if you prefer a more active stretch.
◆ **Recline into a restorative version** for a gentler variation.

Meridians & Elements

Meridian	Element	Function in Pose
Bladder	Water (Yang)	Supports spinal relaxation and forward folding
Kidney	Water (Yin)	Facilitates deep grounding and energy circulation
Liver	Wood (Yin)	Encourages emotional release and hip flexibility

Shoelace Seated/Folded

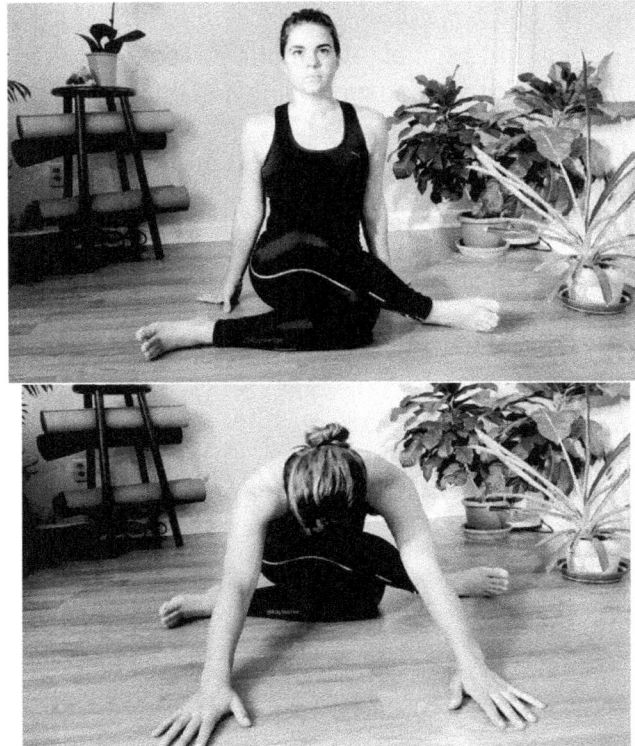

Instructions

1. Begin in **Tabletop Position** (hands and knees).
2. Bring your **right knee forward**, placing it behind your left wrist.
3. **Cradle your left knee behind your right**, stacking them if possible.
4. Sit back between your feet, ensuring they are **wider than your hips** for comfort.
5. Hold for **up to 3 minutes**, breathing into the hips.

Effects

✓ **Stretches piriformis and outer hips**
✓ **Enhances external hip rotation in both legs**
✓ **Provides a deep lower back stretch when folding forward**

Considerations

! **Ankle or knee sensitivity**
! **SI joint discomfort**
! **Limited mobility in hips** ("just won't go" feeling)

Customizations

◆ **Place a blanket or bolster** under the knees for support.
◆ **Let the knees widen** if the pose feels too intense.
◆ **Fold forward** for a deeper low-back stretch, but ensure the spine remains long.
◆ **Take Double Pigeon** (Agnistambhasana) as an alternative.

Meridians & Elements

Meridian	Element	Function in Pose
Liver	Wood (Yin)	Releases emotional tension stored in the hips
Kidney	Water (Yin)	Grounds energy, supporting deep stillness
Gallbladder	Wood (Yang)	Facilitates flexibility and decision-making

Double Pigeon Seated/Folded

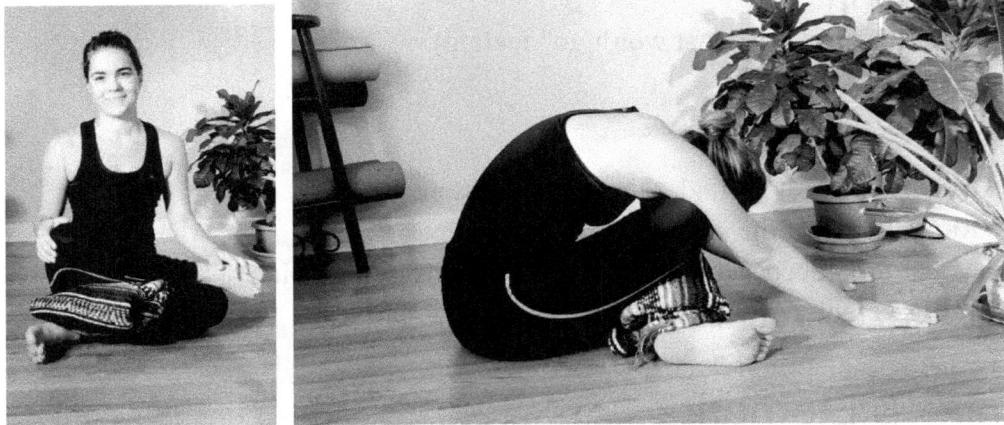

Double Pigeon Pose (Agnistambhasana)

Instructions

1. Begin in **a seated position** with your legs extended forward.
2. Bend your **right knee to create a right angle**, ensuring your thigh is perpendicular to your hip.
3. **Cross your left ankle over your right knee**, stacking the shins on top of each other like logs.
4. Keep your **feet flexed** to protect the knees.
5. Sit **upright** or **fold forward** for a deeper stretch.
6. Hold for **up to 3 minutes**, then switch sides.

Effects

✔ **Deep piriformis stretch**
✔ **Enhances external hip rotation in both legs**
✔ **Releases tension in the lower back when folded forward** (be mindful of sacrum positioning)

Considerations

⚠ **Ankle sensitivity**—avoid excessive pressure on the joint.
⚠ **Knee discomfort**—modify or use props if needed.

Customizations

◆ **Use a blanket or bolster** under the knees for support.
◆ **Let the knees widen** slightly for less intensity.
◆ **Fold forward gently**, maintaining a neutral spine.
◆ **Opt for Shoelace Pose** (Gomukhasana) if this variation is inaccessible.

Meridians & Elements

Meridian	Element	Function in Pose
Liver	Wood (Yin)	Encourages emotional release stored in the hips
Gallbladder	Wood (Yang)	Facilitates lateral movement and flexibility
Kidney	Water (Yin)	Grounds energy, promoting deep rest
Bladder	Water (Yang)	Supports the spine and nervous system

Toes Pose

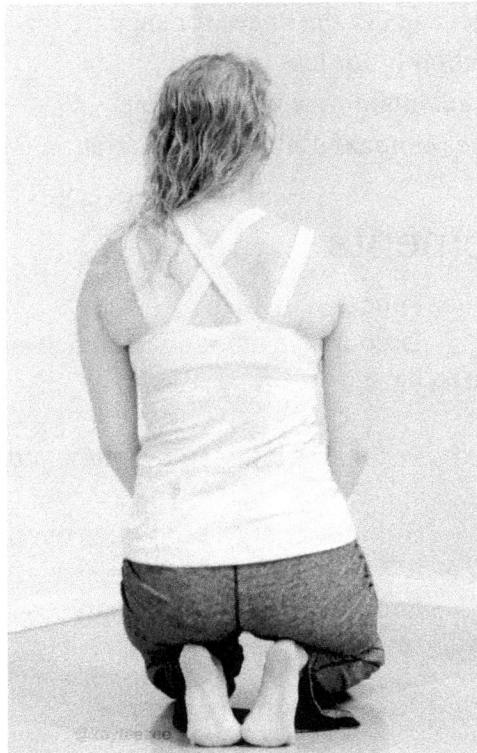

Instructions

1. Begin in **Tabletop Position**, with hands stacked under shoulders and knees under hips.
2. **Tuck your toes under**, keeping the toes spread and aligned.
3. Sit your **hips back onto your heels**, keeping knees in line with your hip bones.
4. Maintain a **neutral spine** and relax the shoulders.
5. Hold for **1-3 minutes**, breathing deeply.

Effects

✓ **Stretches the plantar fascia** and strengthens foot mobility.
✓ **Elongates the quadriceps** and opens the ankle joints.
✓ **Encourages grounding and stability through the lower body.**

Considerations

⚠ **Bunions or toe injuries**—this pose can put pressure on sensitive areas.
⚠ **Metatarsal breaks/stress fractures**—avoid if experiencing acute foot pain.
⚠ **Knee discomfort**—modify or use props if needed.

Customizations

◆ **Lean forward** slightly to reduce intensity.
◆ **Use a rolled blanket or towel** behind the knees for support.
◆ **Skip entirely** if foot structure prevents safe engagement.

Meridians & Elements

Meridian	Element	Function in Pose
Stomach	Earth (Yang)	Stimulates digestion and grounding energy
Bladder	Water (Yin)	Opens the backline of the body, supporting flexibility

Hero's Pose

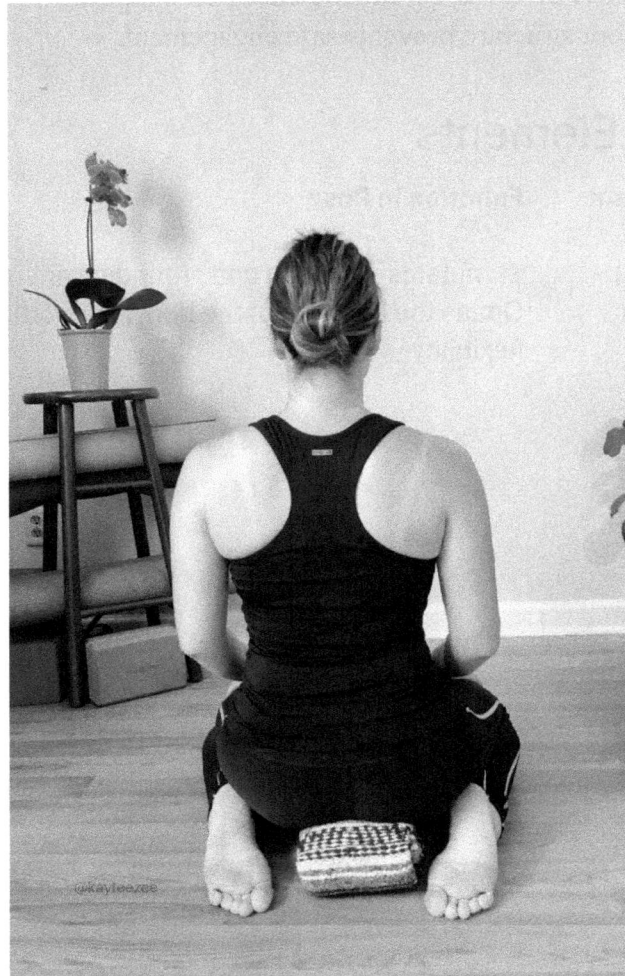

Instructions

1. Start **kneeling** with knees together and feet slightly wider than your hips.
2. Sit back **between your feet**, keeping the tops of the feet pressing into the floor.
3. Keep your **spine upright** and shoulders relaxed.
4. If your **buttocks reach the floor**, you may recline back onto your elbows or all the way down for a deeper stretch.
5. Hold for **up to 3 minutes**, breathing deeply.

Effects

✓ **Stretches the quadriceps** and hip flexors.
✓ **Lengthens the top of the foot** and ankle joints.
✓ **Gently opens the knees**, supporting mobility.
✓ **Deepens into a backbend** if reclining fully.

Considerations

! **Knee pain**—avoid if discomfort is sharp or persistent.
! **Ankle sensitivity**—adjust foot positioning as needed.

Customizations

◆ **Place a block or bolster** under the hips to reduce knee strain.
◆ **Widen the knees** slightly for a more accessible version.
◆ **Tuck a blanket** under the feet for extra ankle support.

Meridians & Elements

Meridian	Element	Function in Pose
Liver	Wood (Yin)	Supports flexibility and emotional flow
Kidney	Water (Yin)	Nourishes endurance and deep restoration
Gall Bladder	Wood (Yang)	Encourages balance and decision-making
Spleen	Earth (Yin)	Grounds and stabilizes energy
Stomach	Earth (Yang)	Strengthens digestion and core integrity

Dragon / Lunge

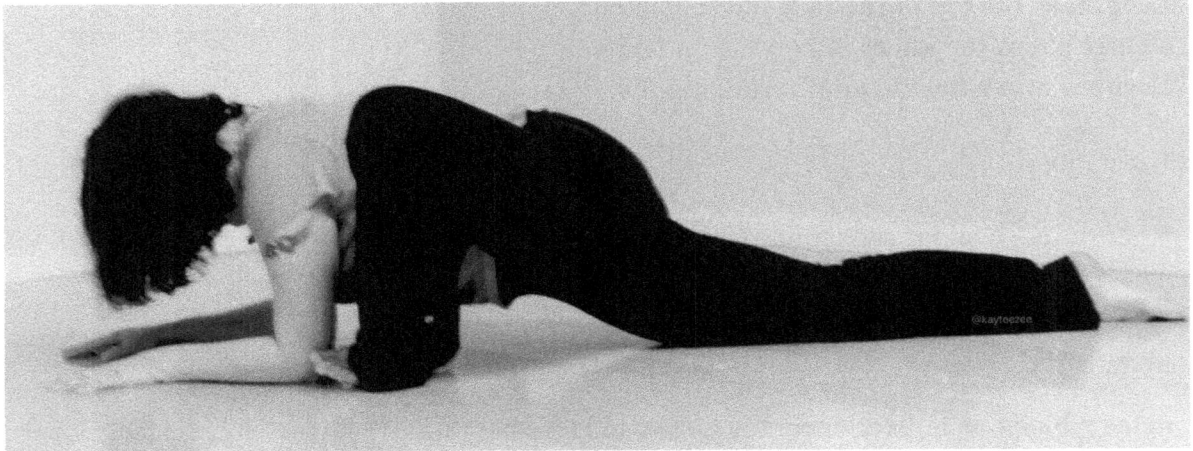

Instructions

1. Start in **Tabletop** (hands and knees).
2. Step your **right foot forward** to the outside of your right hand, keeping your toes pointed forward or slightly turned out.
3. **Slide your left leg back**, extending it fully and lowering your hips toward the floor.
4. Keep your **spine long** and chest open.
5. Hold for **up to 3 minutes**, then switch sides.

Effects

✓ **Deep hip flexor stretch** in the back leg.
✓ **Opens the groin and hip joint** for mobility.
✓ **Stretches the piriformis**, supporting hip stability.
✓ **Encourages external rotation** in the front leg.

Considerations

! **Knee pain**—pad the back knee if needed.
! **Low back discomfort**—engage core for support.
! **Ankle/foot sensitivity**—adjust position as needed.

Customizations

◆ **Support the back knee** with a folded blanket or towel.
◆ **Lower to forearms** for a deeper stretch.

- **Turn front toes out slightly** to ease hip tension.
- **Press the front thigh away from the torso** for a more intense opening.

Meridians & Elements

Meridian	Element	Function in Pose
Liver	Wood (Yin)	Encourages emotional flow and flexibility
Kidney	Water (Yin)	Supports endurance and fluid movement
Stomach	Earth (Yang)	Aids digestion and core grounding
Spleen	Earth (Yin)	Stabilizes and strengthens connective tissues
Gall Bladder	Wood (Yang)	Enhances balance and directional focus

Sleeping Swan / ½ Pigeon

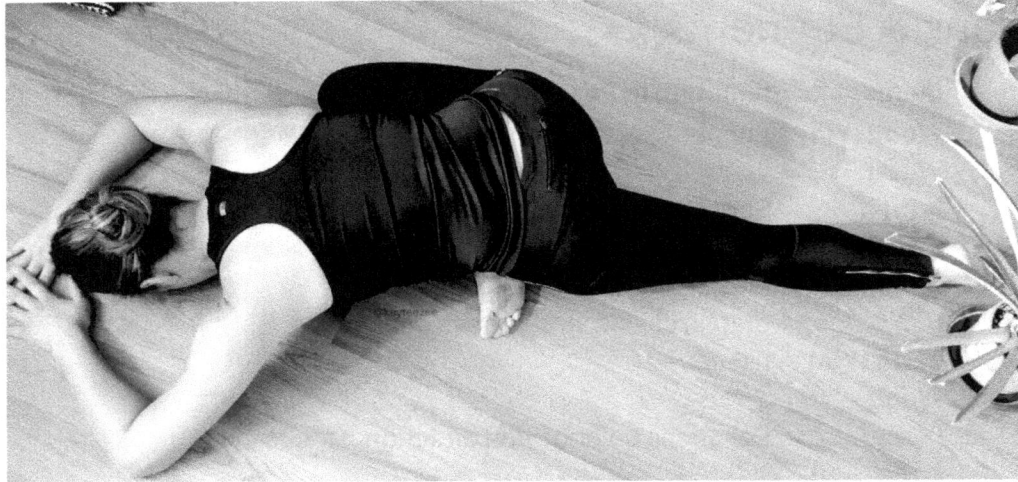

Instructions

1. Start from Tabletop (Downward Dog if it's usual for you)
2. Bring your right knee forward to your right hand and allow the foot to cross towards the left side.
3. Extend the left leg back and fold forward, keeping the pelvis as square as possible.
4. Hold for up to 3 minutes, breathing deeply.

Effects

✓ Stretches the hip flexors of the extended leg.
✓ Deep release for the psoas and piriformis muscles.
✓ Encourages external rotation in the front leg.

Considerations

! Knee pain—modify or use props if discomfort arises.
! Hip pain—ensure even weight distribution.
! Ankle pain—adjust foot positioning to reduce strain.

Customizations

◆ Rest the front leg/hip on a bolster for support.
◆ Place a towel under the back knee for cushioning.
◆ Take Figure 4 variation on the back if pigeon is inaccessible.

Meridians & Elements

Meridian	Element	Function in Pose
Liver	Wood (Yin)	Encourages circulation and emotional release
Kidney	Water (Yin)	Supports grounding and energy flow
Stomach	Earth (Yang)	Assists digestion and stability
Spleen	Earth (Yin)	Enhances nourishment and energy distribution
Gallbladder	Wood (Yang)	Promotes flexibility and lateral movement

Caterpillar Pose

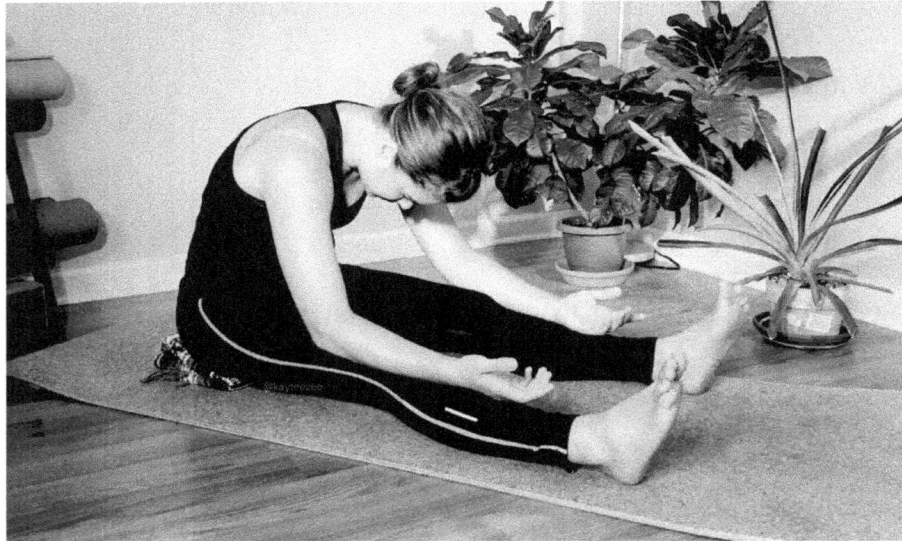

Instructions

1. Sit with your legs extended straight in front of you.
2. Hinge at the hips and fold forward, allowing the spine to gently round.
3. Relax the upper body and let gravity deepen the stretch.
4. Hold for up to 5 minutes, breathing deeply.

Effects

✓ "Keeps abdominal organs free from sluggishness" (Light on Yoga).
✓ Stretches the spine and lengthens the posterior chain.
✓ Compresses the abdomen, stimulating digestion.

Considerations

⚠ Sciatica—modify with props to reduce strain.
⚠ SI joint pain—keep knees slightly bent or avoid deep folding.
⚠ Pregnancy—practice with a wider leg position or avoid deep compression.
⚠ Heartburn—maintain a lifted chest to reduce discomfort.

Customizations

◆ Place a wedge behind the sacrum to lift the pelvis.
◆ Bend or support the knees to ease tension in the lower back.

- Rest the upper body on a bolster for a gentler experience.
- Keep the lower back extended and the chest slightly lifted for more comfort.

Meridians & Elements

Meridian	Element	Function in Pose
Bladder	Water (Yang)	Encourages spinal flexibility and flow of Qi

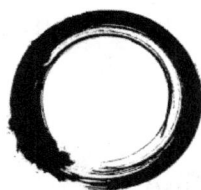

Twists and Side Body

Twists are typically practiced before Savasana to complete the spine's full range of motion, ensuring it moves in all six directions. This is why Banana Pose is included here as well—it gently stretches and elongates the side body, complementing spinal twists for a more balanced and integrated practice.

The twists/side body postures included here are:

Easy Twist

Banana Pose

Twisted Root Twist

Easy Twist

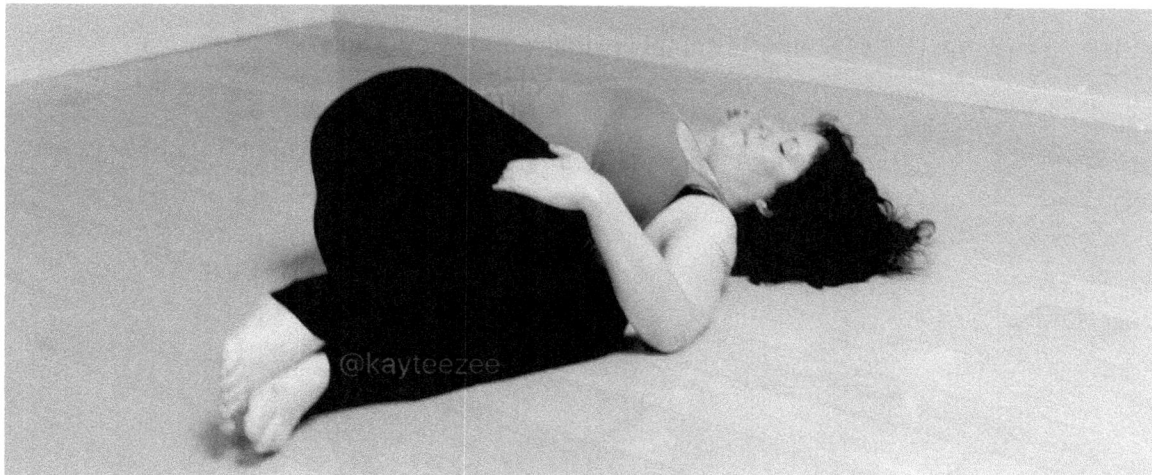

Instructions

1. Lie on your back and bend your knees into your chest.
2. Drop your knees to the right while keeping your shoulders grounded.
3. Extend your left arm to the side, allowing the shoulder to open toward the floor.
4. Keep your neck neutral or gently turn your head to the left.
5. Hold for up to 3 minutes, breathing deeply.
6. Repeat on the other side.

Effects

✓ Gently nurtures the shoulders and upper back.
✓ Provides a mild IT band stretch.
✓ Encourages spinal mobility and relaxation.

Considerations

! SI joint pain—modify by using props or keeping legs staggered.
! GI discomfort—adjust the depth of the twist to avoid compression.

Customizations

◆ Place a towel between the knees for added support.
◆ Use a towel or bolster under the shoulder if it lifts off the floor.
◆ Keep the bottom leg straight and bring the top knee to the chest to minimize sciatic discomfort (Sara Powers modification).

Meridians & Elements

Meridian	Element	Function in Pose
Bladder	Water (Yang)	Supports spinal flexibility and energy flow
Heart	Fire (Yin)	Opens the chest, promoting emotional balance
Lung	Metal (Yin)	Encourages deep breathing and lung expansion

Banana Pose

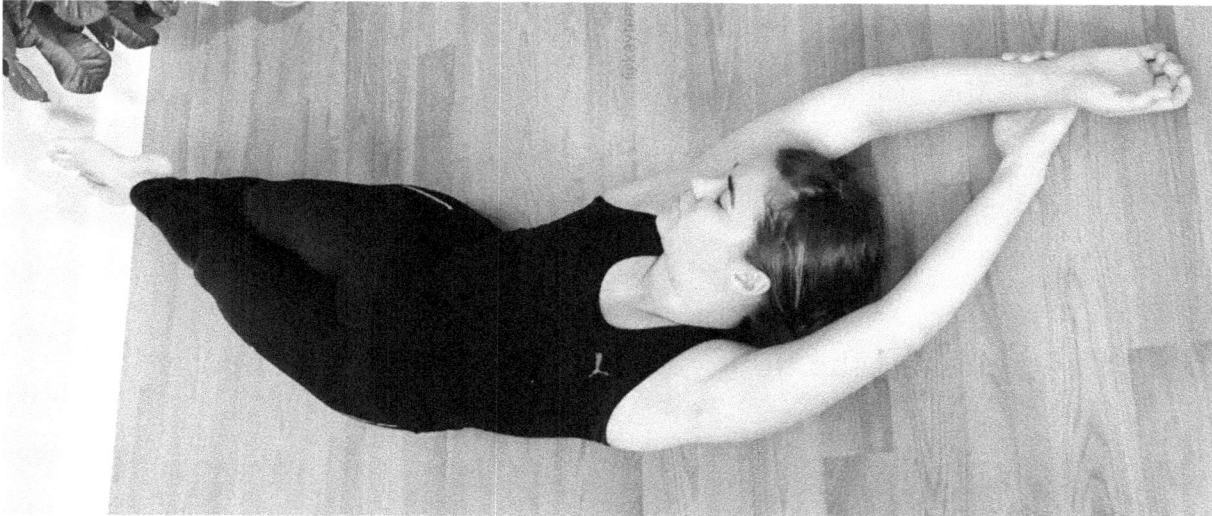

Instructions

Starting on your back, bring your hands above your head, and arch hands and feet towards each other

Keep as much of the back line of your body on the floor as possible

Some practitioners cross the ankles

Keep knees, shoulders and elbows relaxed

Hold for 3-5 minutes

Effects

Stretches lateral line

Mild stretch for IT band

Considerations

Numbness in hands

Shoulder pain

Neck pain

Customizations

Keep arms to the side

Pad the ankles

Small bolster or towel under knees

Bend the elbows

Support the neck

If a shoulder lifts off the floor, you can place a blanket under it

Meridians

Gal Bladder

Heart

Elements

Wood (Yang)

Fire (Yin)

Twisted Root Twist (Forrest)

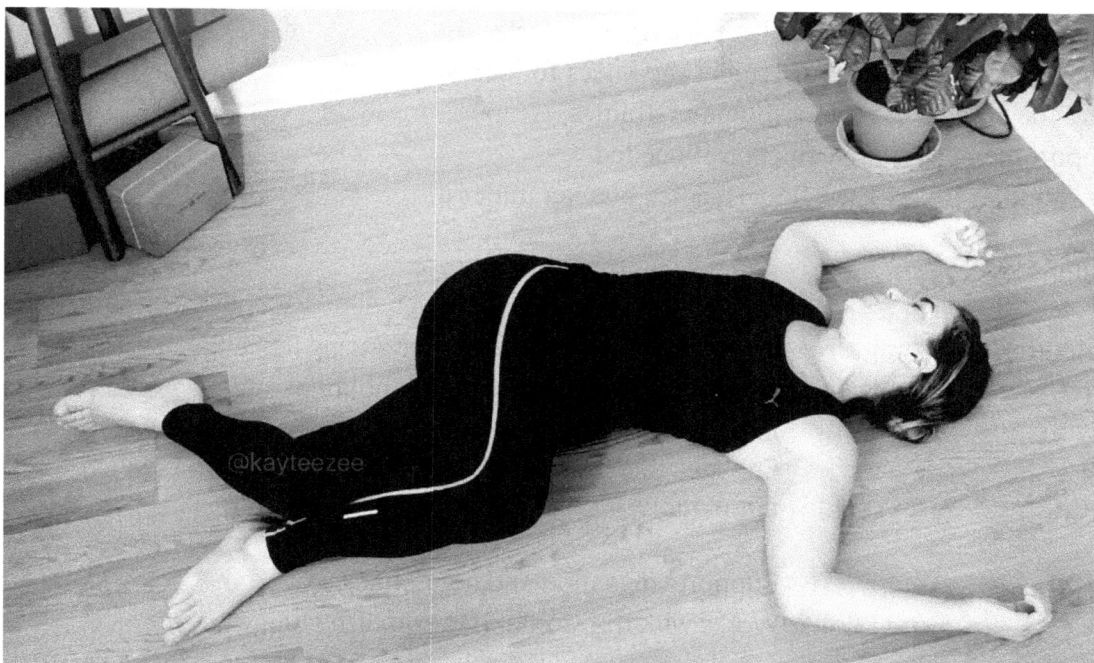

Banana Pose

Instructions

1. Lie on your back and extend your arms overhead.
2. Arch your hands and feet towards each other, creating a crescent shape with your body.
3. Keep as much of the backline of your body on the floor as possible.
4. Optionally, cross the ankles for a deeper stretch.
5. Keep the knees, shoulders, and elbows relaxed.
6. Hold for 3–5 minutes, breathing deeply.

Effects

✓ Stretches the entire lateral line of the body.
✓ Provides a mild stretch for the IT band.
✓ Creates space in the ribcage, promoting deeper breathing.

Considerations

! Numbness in hands—adjust arm position or take breaks if needed.
! Shoulder pain—keep arms lower or modify with props.
! Neck pain—support the head if discomfort arises.

Customizations

◆ Keep arms by the sides if overhead reach is uncomfortable.
◆ Place padding under the ankles for extra comfort.
◆ Use a small bolster or towel under the knees for support.
◆ Bend the elbows to reduce shoulder strain.
◆ Support the neck with a cushion if needed.
◆ If a shoulder lifts off the floor, place a blanket under it.

Meridian	Element	Function in Pose
Gallbladder	Wood (Yang)	Stretches the lateral body, enhancing flexibility
Heart	Fire (Yin)	Opens the chest, supporting emotional release
Lung	Metal (Yin)	Expands the ribcage, deepens breath capacity
Small Intestine	Fire (Yang)	Engages the arms and shoulders, improving circulation
Stomach	Earth (Yang)	Supports digestion and nourishes Qi
Spleen	Earth (Yin)	Works with the stomach to stabilize energy flow

Some Sequences for Your Contemplation:

Peaceful Sequence

(A gentle sequence for nervous system support, heart-opening, and emotional resilience)

1. **Easy Twist** – Encourages spinal mobility and nurtures shoulder release.
2. **Sleeping Swan / Half Pigeon** – Opens the hips and supports emotional grounding.
3. **Caterpillar** – A forward fold that calms the mind and releases tension.
4. **Banana Pose** – Expands the lateral body, allowing for deeper breath and energetic flow.
5. **Savasana with Inner Smile Meditation** – Visualizing a smile filling each organ with warmth and light.

Healing Sounds Sequence

(A posture-based exploration of the Six Healing Sounds, integrating breath, vibration, and meridian activation)

The breaths here are for you to explore for a few rounds. If you are inclined to hold the posture for a bit, you are not obligated to keep the specific breath.

1. **Hugging the Earth (Spleen – "Whooo")** – A deep, grounded fold, connecting to the earth and stabilizing the body's center.
2. **Caterpillar (Lungs – "Sssss")** – A forward fold that compresses the abdomen, supporting the lungs and large intestine.
3. **Easy Twist (Liver – "Shhh")** – Encourages detoxification and emotional release through gentle spinal rotation.
4. **Sleeping Swan / Half Pigeon (Kidneys – "Choo")** – Deeply supports the kidneys, unlocking held fear and fatigue.
5. **Banana Pose (Heart – "Haaa")** – Expands the chest and ribcage, allowing for heart energy and joy to emerge.
6. **Savasana with Sound Integration** – Holding awareness on the vibrational effect of each sound in the body.

Constructive Rest & Backbending Sequence

(A slow, supported approach to backbending that emphasizes release rather than force)

1. **Constructive Rest** – Begin with knees bent, feet on the floor, and hands resting on the belly. Allow the spine to settle into a neutral state.
2. **Banana Pose** – A lateral extension that gently opens the side body and ribs, preparing for deeper expansion.
3. **Sleeping Swan / Half Pigeon** – A hip opener that subtly introduces spinal extension while grounding the lower body.
4. **Supported Fish Pose** – Place a bolster or rolled blanket under the upper back to open the chest and heart. Keep the neck neutral and arms relaxed.
5. **Constructive Rest (Final Return)** – Return to the starting position, allowing the body to absorb the effects of the practice.

Fluid Spinal Unwinding Sequence

(A progression from foundation to release, integrating gentle movement, subtle backbending, and deep rest)

1. **Tabletop** – Establishes a neutral foundation, allowing for awareness of weight and breath.
2. **Cat-Cow** – Creates fluid motion through the spine, preparing for deeper release.
3. **Thread the Needle** – A gentle twist to open the shoulders and upper back.
4. **Puppy Pose** – Extends the spine while softening the chest toward the earth.
5. **Sphinx Pose** – A subtle backbend that gently awakens the front body.
6. **Hugging the Earth** – Grounds and integrates, surrendering tension into the floor.
7. **Flip to Back** – Transition smoothly while keeping awareness on spinal alignment.
8. **Banana Pose** – Expands the lateral body, creating space and balance.
9. **Savasana** – Complete stillness, absorbing the effects of the practice.

Legs Up the Wall with the Six Healing Sounds

(A deeply restorative sequence combining inversion with vibrational healing)

1. **Set Up in Legs Up the Wall** – Lie on your back with legs resting against the wall, allowing the spine to settle. Arms can be at the sides, on the belly, or overhead. Focus on slow, steady breathing.
2. **Begin the Healing Sounds:**
   - **Lungs ("Sssss")** – Exhale ssss, expanding the ribcage and releasing tension from the chest.
   - **Kidneys ("Choo")** – Exhale choo, directing awareness to the lower back and softening the kidneys.
   - **Liver ("Shhh")** – Exhale shhh, releasing stored frustration and allowing the side body to open.
   - **Heart ("Haaa")** – Exhale haaa, vibrating warmth and spaciousness into the chest.
   - **Spleen ("Whooo")** – Exhale whooo, grounding energy into the center of the body.
   - **Triple Burner ("Heeee")** – Exhale heeee, balancing and integrating the full system.
3. **Stillness in Legs Up the Wall** – Remain in the posture for several minutes, allowing the energy to settle and flow naturally. Let the breath return to a soft, effortless rhythm.
4. **Savasana Transition** – Slowly slide away from the wall and rest flat, absorbing the effects of sound, stillness, and inversion.

Conclusion: The Return to Resonance

This work is not a theory. It is not a system to memorize or a framework to impose. It is a **way of perceiving, sensing, and attuning to what has always been present.** From the **Five Phases to the Extraordinary Vessels, from the Immortals to the neuroaffective field of embodied experience**, every chapter in this book has been an invitation—an opening rather than a closing. Each map is a lens, each structure a possibility, each pattern a movement waiting to be felt.

At the core of this journey is **resonance, not force.** Healing, transformation, and cognition do not happen through dominance, but through alignment—**through the ways we learn to listen, to integrate, to move with rather than against.**

What This Means in Practice

- **Your body is not broken.** Trauma is not damage—it is an imprint, a pattern, a rhythm that can be re-tuned.
- **Your nervous system is an orienting system, not a regulation system.** It is not about controlling your state—it is about learning how state emerges from gravity, fascia, perception, and lineage.
- **Your experience is valid.** Healing is not about returning to an imposed definition of "normal"—it is about moving into deeper coherence with what is actually happening inside you.
- **You are already inside the system.** The tools, the knowledge, the pathways—all of it is already present. This is not about adding more, but about noticing what has been moving beneath the surface all along.

The Path Forward

This book is a starting point, not a conclusion. The goal was never to give you answers, but to give you **the right questions**—questions that open doors rather than closing them.

What happens next is yours to explore.

- What would it feel like to move with curiosity rather than control?
- What if healing was not about fixing, but about **re-patterning**?
- What if consciousness was not something you "have," but something you **participate in**?

The work does not end with this book. It moves through your breath, your body, your awareness.

It moves **through the Soma → to the Self.**
It moves **through the Soma → to the Spirit.**
It moves **through the Soma → to the World.**

This is where we step beyond theory. This is where it becomes lived.

This is where the next spiral begins.

Bibliography:

Books

Chace, C. (2021). An exposition of the eight extraordinary vessels: Acupuncture, alchemy, and herbal medicine. London: Singing Dragon.

Chia, M. (1993). Awaken healing energy of the Tao. Healing Tao Books.

Lesondak, D. (2017). Fascia: What it is and why it matters. Handspring Publishing.

Manne, K. (2020). Entitled: How male privilege hurts women. New York: Crown.

Menakem, R. (2021). The quaking of America: An embodied guide to navigating our nation's upheaval and racial reckoning. Las Vegas: Central Recovery Press.

Netter, F. H. (2018). Atlas of human anatomy (7th ed.). Philadelphia: Elsevier.

Panksepp, J., & Biven, L. (2012). The archaeology of mind: Neuroevolutionary origins of human emotions. New York: W. W. Norton & Company.

Porges, S. W. (2011). The polyvagal theory: Neurophysiological foundations of emotions, attachment, communication, and self-regulation. New York: W. W. Norton.

Pregadio, F. (2019). Taoist internal alchemy: An anthology of Neidan texts. Mountain View, CA: Golden Elixir Press.

Rossi, E. (2007). Shen: Psycho-emotional aspects of Chinese medicine. Churchill Livingstone Elsevier.

Tufte, E. R. (1983). The visual display of quantitative information. Cheshire, CT: Graphics Press.

Unschuld, P. U. (2011). (Trans.) The Yellow Emperor's classic of medicine: A new translation of the Neijing Suwen with commentary. Boston & London: Shambhala.

Book Chapters

Pregadio, F. (2016). Creation and its inversion: Cosmos, human being, and elixir in the Cantong Qi (The Seal of the Unity of the Three). In A. Andreeva & D. Steavu (Eds.), Transforming the void: Embryological discourse and reproductive imagery in East Asian religions (pp. 139–162). Leiden: Brill.

Reports

Substance Abuse and Mental Health Services Administration (SAMHSA). (2014). SAMHSA's concept of trauma and guidance for a trauma-informed approach. Rockville, MD: U.S. Department of Health and Human Services.

Collaborative Works

Chace, A. D., Duncan, & Leitch, L. (2019). The Tao of trauma: A practitioner's guide for integrating five element theory and trauma treatment. North Atlantic Books.

Washington, H. A. (2006). Medical apartheid: The dark history of medical experimentation on Black Americans from colonial times to the present. Doubleday.

Nervous System Regulation

- **Polyvagal Theory)**
    - ○ Developed by **Stephen Porges**, this theory explains how the **autonomic nervous system (ANS)** regulates safety, connection, and defense states.
    - ○ **Key insight:** The ANS does not just respond to threats—it constantly scans for **cues of safety or danger**, a process called **Neuroception** (see below).
    - ○ **Cross-reference:** Shen, Qi, Wu Wei, Afferent/Efferent, Vagus Nerve, Fascia
- **Neuroception – "Sensing Before Thinking"**
    - ○ The **body detects** safety or threat **before conscious awareness**.
    - ○ This is why **regulation cannot be forced**—it emerges from **the environment, movement, and breath.**
    - ○ **Cross-reference:** Afferent vs. Efferent, Tensegrity, Wu Wei
- **The Three Polyvagal States:**
    - ○ **Ventral Vagal State: "Safe & Secure"**
        - ▪ The **social engagement** system. Safe, open, curious.
        - ▪ **Aligned with:** The Pericardium & Heart meridians, Shen, Wu Wei.
    - ○ **Sympathetic Activation "Mobilized, Fight-or-Flight"**
        - ▪ The **active defense** system. Alert, reactive, ready to move.
        - ▪ **Aligned with:** Liver & Gallbladder meridians, Yang Wei Mai.
    - ○ **Dorsal Vagal Shutdown – "Collapsed & Frozen"**
        - ▪ The **immobilization** system. Numb, withdrawn, shut down.
        - ▪ **Aligned with:** Kidney & Bladder meridians, Yin Wei Mai.
- **Afferent vs. Efferent**
    - ○ **Afferent signals** (incoming) carry information **from the body to the brain** → Shen perceives first.
    - ○ **Efferent signals** (outgoing) carry information **from the brain to the body** → Action follows awareness.
    - ○ **Cross-reference:** Shen, Qi, Fascia, Sensorimotor Experience
- **Regulation vs. Resonance**
    - ○ **Regulation** = Returning to balance within oneself.
    - ○ **Resonance** = Achieving balance **through connection**—with people, movement, and the environment.
    - ○ **Key insight: We do not "self-regulate" in isolation—our nervous system relies on resonance.**
- **The Vagus Nerve The "Body-Mind Connector"**
    - ○ A massive nerve regulating **breath, digestion, heart rate, and social engagement.**
    - ○ **Why it matters:**
        - ▪ Engages **both parasympathetic (rest/digest) and sympathetic (fight/flight) functions**.
        - ▪ Can be **toned** through breath, vocalization, and gentle movement.
    - ○ **Cross-reference:** Neuroception, Yin & Yang Balance, Extraordinary Vessels, Shen

Tensegrity & Wu Wei in the Body

- **Tensegrity – "Tensional Integrity"**
  - A structural principle where **stability emerges from balance between tension & compression.**
  - The **body is not a stack of bones**—it is a **dynamic web of forces.**
  - **Cross-reference:** Fascia, Wu Wei, Sensorimotor Experience
- **Fascia– "The Living Matrix"**
  - A **continuous connective tissue network** that holds the body's shape.
  - Fascia **does not just store trauma—it organizes movement, posture, and sensory perception.**
  - **Cross-reference:** Extraordinary Vessels, Sensorimotor Experience
- **Wu Wei in the Body– "Effortless Movement"**
  - Moving **without unnecessary tension**—allowing action to arise naturally.
  - This is **not passive**—it is the cultivation of **functional adaptability.**
  - **Cross-reference:** Tensegrity, Polyvagal Theory, Shen, Qi
- **The Three Planes of Motion:**
  - **Sagittal – Forward & Backward (Shen, Water)**
  - **Coronal– Side-to-Side (Qi, Fire)**
  - **Transverse – Rotational (Jing, Earth)**
  - **Cross-reference:** Neijing Tu, Sensorimotor Experience, Meridians

Daoism & Internal Alchemy (Neidan – 內丹, Nèidān)

- **Dao (道, Dào) – "The Way"**
  - The fundamental principle of natural order, balance, and effortless flow. Everything arises from and returns to Dao.
  - **See also:** Wu Wei, Qi, Shen
- **Jing (精, Jīng) – Essence**
  - The densest, most material aspect of life force, stored in the Kidneys. It governs genetics, growth, and vitality.
  - **See also:** Qi, Shen, Extraordinary Vessels
- **Qi (氣, Qì) – Vital Energy**
  - The movement of life force, connecting body, mind, and environment. Qi circulates through the meridians and governs physiological and energetic function.
  - **See also:** Jing, Shen, Meridians
- **Shen (神, Shén) – Spirit, Consciousness**
  - The most refined aspect of Qi, associated with perception, wisdom, and awareness. Each organ has its own Shen.
  - **See also:** Organ Shen, Neijing Tu, Extraordinary Vessels
- **Neidan (內丹, Nèidān) – Internal Alchemy**
  - The Daoist practice of refining Jing, Qi, and Shen for transformation. Unlike external alchemy (Waidan), which focuses on elixirs, Neidan is an internal process of cultivating energy and perception.

- o **See also:** Extraordinary Vessels, Shen, Wu Wei
- **Wu Wei (無為, Wú Wéi) – Effortless Action**
  - o The practice of moving in alignment with natural forces rather than forcing outcomes. It is the foundation of **spontaneous, embodied wisdom**.
  - o **See also:** Dao, Neidan, Tensegrity

The Eight Trigrams (八卦, Bāguà)

(Fundamental forces shaping consciousness, body function, and natural patterns.)

Trigram	Pinyin	Element	Direction	Attributes
☰ Qián	Qián	Metal	Northwest	Strength, leadership, clarity
☷ Kūn	Kūn	Earth	Southwest	Receptivity, nourishment, stability
☳ Zhèn	Zhèn	Wood	East	Activation, movement, boldness
☴ Xùn	Xùn	Wood	Southeast	Expansion, wisdom, inheritance
☵ Kǎn	Kǎn	Water	North	Depth, emotion, adaptability
☶ Gèn	Gèn	Earth	Northeast	Stillness, vision, endurance
☲ Lí	Lí	Fire	South	Illumination, transformation, passion
☱ Duì	Duì	Metal	West	Joy, expression, spontaneity

See also: Five Elements, Extraordinary Vessels, Body Bagua

The Twelve Primary Meridians (經絡, Jīngluò)

Meridian	Pinyin	Element	Paired Organ	Primary Function
Lung	*Fèi Jīng*	Metal	Large Intestine	Respiration, grief processing
Large Intestine	*Dàcháng Jīng*	Metal	Lung	Elimination, boundary-setting
Stomach	*Wèi Jīng*	Earth	Spleen	Digestion, assimilation of nourishment
Spleen	*Pí Jīng*	Earth	Stomach	Blood production, grounding energy
Heart	*Xīn Jīng*	Fire	Small Intestine	Joy, Shen (spirit) consciousness
Small Intestine	*Xiǎocháng Jīng*	Fire	Heart	Sorting truth from illusion
Bladder	*Pángguāng Jīng*	Water	Kidney	Fluid movement, fear release
Kidney	*Shèn Jīng*	Water	Bladder	Jing storage, longevity, willpower
Pericardium	*Xīnbāo Jīng*	Fire	Triple Burner	Heart protection, emotional stability
Triple Burner	*Sānjiāo Jīng*	Fire	Pericardium	Metabolism, thermoregulation
Liver	*Gān Jīng*	Wood	Gallbladder	Vision, emotional flow
Gallbladder	*Dǎn Jīng*	Wood	Liver	Decision-making, courage

(Organ-energy systems that regulate bodily functions and emotional states.)

See also: Extraordinary Vessels, Five Elements, Organ Shen

Organ Shen

Organ	Shen)	Function	Emotional & Psychological Role	Element
Heart (心, Xīn)	Shen (神)	Governs consciousness, awareness, and perception	Clarity, wisdom, love, and connection; imbalance can cause anxiety, restlessness, or scattered thoughts	Fire 🔥
Liver (肝, Gān)	Hun (魂)	Stores vision, purpose, and dreams	Governs creativity, long-term planning, and intuition; imbalance may lead to frustration, indecisiveness, or feeling stuck	Wood 🌳
Spleen (脾, Pí)	Yi (意)	Manages thought, focus, and intellect	Supports memory, learning, and grounded thinking; imbalance can cause worry, overthinking, or mental fatigue	Earth 🌍
Lungs (肺, Fèi)	Po (魄)	Governs primal instincts, body awareness, and breath	Regulates deep presence, survival instincts, and grief processing; imbalance may lead to disconnection, sadness, or difficulty letting go	Metal ⛰
Kidneys (肾, Shèn)	Zhi (志)	Governs willpower, stamina, and resilience	Provides determination, perseverance, and deep inner strength; imbalance can cause fear, lack of motivation, or burnout	Water 💧

IV. The Eight Extraordinary Vessels (奇經八脈, Qí Jīng Bā Mài)

(Deep channels regulating **postural patterns, developmental structure, and embodied memory.**)

Vessel	Pinyin	Element	Function
Du Mai (Governing)	Dū Mài	Metal	Yang energy, spine, willpower
Ren Mai (Conception)	Rèn Mài	Earth	Yin energy, nourishment, self-compassion
Chong Mai (Penetrating)	Chōng Mài	Fire	Ancestral memory, transformation
Dai Mai (Belt)	Dài Mài	Earth	Core stability, inherited patterns
Yang Wei Mai (Yang Linking)	Yáng Wéi Mài	Wood	External adaptability, dynamic response
Yin Wei Mai (Yin Linking)	Yīn Wéi Mài	Water	Emotional processing, resilience
Yang Qiao Mai (Yang Heel)	Yáng Qiāo Mài	Metal	Action, physical confidence
Yin Qiao Mai (Yin Heel)	Yīn Qiāo Mài	Water	Rest, sleep, subconscious healing

See also: Neidan, Body Bagua, Sensorimotor Experience

V. The Eight Immortals (八仙, Bāxiān)

(Mythic archetypes representing paths of spiritual mastery.)

Immortal	Pinyin	Symbol	Archetype
Lü Dongbin	*Lǚ Dòngbīn*	Sword	Scholar-Sage, Inner Alchemy
He Xiangu	*Hé Xiāngū*	Lotus	Maiden of Health, Feminine Wisdom
Zhang Guolao	*Zhāng Guǒlǎo*	Drum	Mystic Alchemist, Unconventional Wisdom
Lan Caihe	*Lán Cǎihé*	Flowers	Androgynous Wanderer, Impermanence
Zhongli Quan	*Zhōnglí Quán*	Fan	General-Healer, Transformation
Cao Guojiu	*Cáo Guójiù*	Jade Tablet	Noble Patron, Structure
Han Xiangzi	*Hán Xiāngzi*	Flute	Musician, Joyful Resonance
Li Tieguai	*Lǐ Tiěguǎi*	Iron Crutch	Compassionate Wanderer, Resilience

See also: Neidan, Shen, Extraordinary Vessels

www.ingramcontent.com/pod-product-compliance
Lightning Source LLC
Chambersburg PA
CBHW080133270326
41926CB00021B/4458